MINDFUL EATING: STOP OVEREATING AND AVOID BINGE EATING, THE ANTI-DIET FOR LONG TERM WEIGHT-LOSS

TRANSFORM EMOTIONAL EATING TO A HEALTHIER RELATIONSHIP WITH THE FOODS YOU LOVE AND ENJOY

JULIA MEADOWS

ABOUT THE AUTHOR

Julia Meadows is a senior life coach and Wellness expert at the WellnessMastership.com, a life coaching business based in London, England.

Wellness Mastership teaches clients on consciousness, lifting your vibration, the real law of attraction (updated), and the art of living a better life. Through our teaching we have helped clients worldwide gain a better advantage, and help develop themselves and achieve more from want they desire.

We're in the changing lives business.

SCAN ME FOR A BONUS

https://bonus.mindsetmastership.com/mindful-eating

DON'T MISS THIS! YOUR GUIDE TO INCREASING SELF-CONFIDENCE

Introducing *Growing Your Self-Confidence*.

This short but powerful eBook covers a wide range of topics to help you breakthrough your self-doubts, overcome common challenges, build your self-esteem, and unlock your potential:

IN THIS FREE BONUS GUIDE DISCOVER:

- Building Confidence and Self-Esteem
- The Roots of Low Self-Confidence
- How to Boost your Self-Confidence
- And more...

PLUS BONUS NEW FREE BOOK RELEASES!

SCAN THE QR CODE TO CLAIM YOUR FREE BONUS NOW!

https://bonus.mindsetmastership.com/mindful-eating

WANT A COPY OF MY NEW EBOOK?

Email me:
juliameadowsauthor@gmail.com

"Wherever you go, go with all your heart."
— **Confucius**

MASTERSHIP BOOKS

UK | USA | Canada | Ireland | Australia
India | New Zealand | South Africa | China

Mastership Books is part of the United Arts Publishing House group of
companies based in London, England, UK.
First published by Mastership Books (London, UK), 2021
Text Copyright © United Arts Publishing

Cover design by Rich © United Arts Publishing (UK)
Text and internal design by Rich © United Arts Publishing (UK)

Image credits reserved.
Colour separation by Spitting Image Design Studio

Printed and bound in Great Britain
National Publications Association of Britain
London, England, United Kingdom.

Paper design UAP
A723.5

Title: Mindful Eating

Design, Bound & Printed:
London, England,
Great Britain.

Change Mindset Books

GET A FREE AUDIOBOOK

EMAIL SUBJECT LINE:

"MINDFUL EATING"

TO

juliameadowsauthor@gmail.com

CONTENTS

INTRODUCTION

Vitamins, minerals, or molecules are not one of the essential building blocks of dietary metabolism. It's our food friendship, the total of our innermost emotions and ideas on what we consume. This food relationship is as profound and revealing as we might ever have. The great Sufi poet Rumi once remarked: "When they look at a loaf of bread, the satisfied man and the hungry man do not see the same thing." "When I sell liquor, it's called bootlegging," noted gangster Al Capone astutely observed. it's called hospitality when my patrons serve it on silver trays on Lake Shore Drive." Indeed, how we think about food is so profoundly relative that I am connected to it.

Say we were inspecting a plate of pasta, chicken, and salad, for instance. You might see calories and fat in a woman who wants to lose weight. She would react to the salad or chicken favorably, but she would be afraid to look at the pasta. When an athlete is trying to build muscle, she may focus on the chicken and ignore the other foods in a meal because it contains protein. A pure vegetarian can see the gross sight of a dead animal and touch nothing on the plate.

Conversely, a chicken farmer will be proud to see a good piece of meat. Depending on whether or not the plate of food is acceptable on her chosen diet, anyone seeking to cure a disease by diet will see either potential medication or potential poison. A researcher researching food nutrient quality will see a range of chemicals.

Dear Reader,

As independent authors, it's often difficult to gather reviews compared with much bigger publishers.

Therefore, please leave a review on the platform where you bought this book.

KINDLE:

LEAVE A REVIEW HERE < click here >

Many thanks,

Author Team

FINDING BALANCE & NOT BINGE EATING

E arly life growth sets the stage for later development and can affect the susceptibility of individuals to disease. Early life growth should also be taken into account in the personalization of nutrition for mental health. During early brain development, any results of dietary intervention (the so-called first 1000 days, e.g., from conception to 2 years of age) may have a more significant impact on later health than later life interventions. Increasing fundamental understanding of how nutrients influence signaling processes that are important for brain functions would also make progress.

The general functions of the brain include metabolic, endocrine, immune, and other signaling processes, all of which are mediated by the gut microbiota.

The brain accounts for about 13 percent of lean body weight in newborns, and its further growth and development are subject to energy and nutritional constraints. Reliable access to a sufficient dietary supply is necessary during this time of rapid development. The cognitive impairments triggered by early-life malnutrition have been a major focus in nutritional psychiatry. Early-life diet has been shown to influence cognitive performance later in life in rodents and humans.

In addition, groups that are vulnerable to an elevated risk of neurological impairment, such as preterm-born infants or small-term-born infants of gestational age, encourage a clear correlation between nutritional status and the risk of neurological impairment.

All nutrients are necessary for brain development, but long-chain polyunsaturated fatty acids, protein, iron, choline, folate, and vitamins A, D, B6, and B12 are particularly important for neurodevelopment. Experimental studies have shown that the cytoarchitecture of the cerebral cortex during fetal development can be irreversibly disrupted by iodine deficiency. And it induces irregular migratory neuron patterns associated with children with cognitive disabilities. Iron deficiency anemia during infancy is associated with brain connectivity changes, but it has also been shown that the reverse has occurred. More subtle dietary changes may also influence the early development of the brain. Breast milk supplies lipids and, more precisely, omega-3 and 6 polyunsaturated fatty acids DHA (docosahexaenoic acid) and ARA (arachidonic acid), but their concentrations in breast milk are influenced by the mother's dietary intake.

Researchers using mice found that the absorption of omega-3 fatty acids into neuronal membranes was positively affected by a diet enriched with omega-3 fatty acids or reduced omega-6 fatty acid levels. Such a low omega-6 diet has also recently been shown to entirely abolish cognitive impairments caused by early life stress in adult mice. Recent research has shown an increase in cognitive habits and plasticity markers in the adolescent brain in rats exposed to a diet supplemented with omega-3 polyunsaturated fatty acids, eicosapentaenoic acid, docosahexaenoic acid, and docosapentaenoic acid and vitamin A following psychological stress.

The long-term effects of early-life stress were alleviated by the dietary intervention of the milk fat globule membrane (MFGM) and the pre-biotic blend of poly-dextrose/galactic-oligo-saccharide using a rat maternal separation model.

These results illustrate the essential role of a healthy diet in providing a sufficient supply of nutrients to sustain brain growth for later cognitive function and the importance of early life development to (later) psychiatric disease susceptibility, which could explain, at least in part, the variability of treatment effects observed.

What's impressive is that, in reaction to her particular feelings, these eaters will metabolize this same meal very differently. In other words, a food's nutritional value and effect on body weight can be determined by your thoughts and feelings about it, possibly even more so than by the nutrients themselves.

2

HOW THE BRAIN EATS

The brain, spinal cord, and nerves data highway are like a telephone system interacting with your digestive organs through your mind. Let's say you're about to eat a cone of ice cream. In the upper center of the brain-the cerebral cortex-the idea and picture of that ice cream exists. From there, data is electrochemically relayed to the limbic system, known as the "lower" part of the brain. Emotions and main physiological functions such as starvation, hunger, temperature, sex drive, heart rate, and blood pressure are regulated by the limbic system. The limbic system, which unites the mind's actions with the body's biology, contains a pea-sized group of tissues known as the hypothalamus.

In other words, it takes visual, emotional, and thoughtful feedback and translates this data into physiological responses. It's nothing short of a miracle here.

The hypothalamus can modulate this positive feedback by transmitting stimulation signals to the salivary glands, esophagus, stomach, intestines, pancreas, liver, and gallbladder through parasympathetic nerve fibers if the ice cream is your favorite flavor, say, chocolate, and you eat it with a full measure of delight. It will facilitate digestion, resulting in a more thorough metabolic breakdown of the ice cream and more efficient utilization of its caloric content.

If you feel guilty about eating the ice cream or criticize yourself for eating it, with this negative feedback, the hypothalamus will send signals to the sympathetic autonomic nervous system fibers. As a result, the digestive system produces inhibitory reactions, ensuring that the ice cream will be consumed but not fully metabolized.

It might stay longer in your digestive system, reducing the number of beneficial gut bacteria and increasing the release of harmful byproducts into the bloodstream. Additionally, by causing your insulin and cortisol levels to rise, inhibitory signals in your nervous system will reduce your capacity to burn calories, which will cause you to store more of your guilt-inducing ice cream as body fat. As a result, your body immediately experiences what you think about the food you eat, thanks to the central nervous system.

The brain does not discriminate between an actual stressor and an imaginary one. If you were alone, content, and thinking about the person who had wronged you years earlier, and if that incident still has meaning for you, your body would quickly enter the physiological stress state, which is characterized by increased heart rate and blood pressure along with decreased digestive function.

The brain considers any guilt about food, shame about the body, or judgment about health to be stressors and is immediately transformed into its electrochemical equivalents in the body. You can eat the healthiest meal on the planet, but your food digestion goes down, and your fat storage metabolism increases if you think of toxic thoughts. Similarly, you could consume a nutritionally challenged meal, but the nutritious power of your food would be enhanced if your head and heart were in the proper position.

Let's reexamine one of science's most compelling phenomena, the placebo effect, in order to fully comprehend the influence of the mind over metabolism.

In 1983, a new chemotherapy treatment was being tested by medical researchers. A placebo, an artificially produced harmless, inert chemical substance, was administered to the other group of cancer patients in place of the experimental drug. As you might know, to assess the true efficacy of the essence in question, pharmaceutical companies are forced by law to test all potential products against a placebo. Nobody in this study gave it a second thought that one of chemotherapy's most common side effects, hair loss, affected 74% of cancer patients receiving the drug. However, quite remarkably, 31% of the placebo chemotherapy patients-an inert saltwater injection also had an odd side effect: they also lost their hair. The power of expectation is such. The only explanation for losing their hair to those placebo patients is that they thought they would. They associated chemotherapy with going bald, like many individuals.

What do you think happens when we tell ourselves things like, "This cake is fattening? I really shouldn't be eating it," "I'm going to eat this fried chicken, but I know it's bad for me," or "I enjoy eating my salad because it's healthy." If the power of the mind is strong enough to make our hair fall out when taking a placebo, then what do you think happens when we do that?

It's not saying that if we believe it's good for us, we can eat poison without any harm. What we think about the material we eat can have a powerful effect on how it affects the body. Millions of people eat and drink daily while thinking about their meals with clear and compelling feelings.

Consider some of the foods to which you have good links:

- "Salt's going to increase my blood pressure."
- "Fat is going to make me fatter."
- "Sugar is going to rot my teeth." "Without my cup of coffee, I can't make it through the day."
- "This meat will raise my level of cholesterol."
- "My bones will build this calcium."

Some of these statements may be true to a certain degree. Could it be that we are causing these effects? And if these impacts are the inevitable product of eating these foods, do you see how we can change those outcomes with the power of our expectations?

Its type is very commonplace. Researchers have estimated that 35 to 45 percent of all prescription medicines can owe their efficacy to the power of placebo and that 67 percent of all over-the-counter medicines are also focused placeboes, such as headache remedies, cough medicines, and appetite suppressants. The placebo response in some studies is as high as 90 percent.

Amazingly, very few have made the apparent connection between placebo power and food in the scientific community. The placebo effect is, therefore, integrated into the nutritional process. On a day-to-day basis, it's intensely present every time we eat, and it's like phoning your inner dietary pharmacy in a prescription.

What we assume, through nerve pathways, the endocrine system, the circulation of neuropeptides, the immune network, and the digestive tract, is alchemically translated into the body.

CAN FOOD REALLY IMPACT MENTAL HEALTH?

Many individuals are attempting to use self-help to regain care of their mental health and find ways to use it alongside or even instead of prescription medicine. One approach for self-help is to improve what we consume, and there is growing interest in how food and nutrition can influence emotional and mental well-being.

Scientific evidence is emerging to support this, but scientists have several obstacles to address. In the meantime, some medical practitioners must be convinced of the relationship between food and mood. Nevertheless, the value of food and nutrition for preserving or enhancing their emotional and mental health is demonstrated by supportive feedback from people who have improved their diet.

How mood is influenced by food?

The cause-and-effect relationship between food and mood has many theories. Some instances are the following:

- Blood sugar level variations are correlated with mood and energy changes caused by what we eat.
- Brain chemicals affect how we think, sound, and act (neurotransmitters, such as serotonin, dopamine, and acetylcholine).
- They might be influenced by what we have eaten.
- Abnormal reactions, such as artificial colorings and flavorings, to artificial chemicals in foods may occur.
- Some reactions may be due to an enzyme deficiency necessary to digest food. For example, lactase is required to digest lactose (milk sugar); without it, you can build up a milky intolerance.
- Individuals may become food hypersensitive. This can cause what is known as food allergies or sensitivities that are delayed or concealed.
- Inadequate levels of vitamins, minerals, and essential fatty acids can affect mental health, and certain symptoms are linked to particular nutritional deficiencies. Relations between low levels of certain B vitamins and symptoms of schizophrenia, low levels of the mineral zinc and eating disorders, and low levels of omega-3 oils and depression have been shown, for instance.

4

THE PSYCHOLOGICAL CONNECTION
OF FOOD & THE MIND

Generally, it is agreed that how we feel will affect what we eat or drink (mood to food). What needs to be better understood is how our eating will impact our mental functioning (food to mood). One example of a dynamic relationship is the use of caffeine. Caffeine is the world's most commonly used behavior-modifying substance in tea, coffee, cola, and chocolate beverages. If we are tired and irritable, we always prefer to drink it because it can lift us and help us focus. There are also several positive psychological associations with enjoying a cup of coffee or tea. Sitting down with a cup of tea, we meet a friend for 'coffee and a chat' or give ourselves a break, which is essential. But too much caffeine can cause symptoms such as anxiety, nervousness, and depression (which is a different amount for each of us). Any diet and mood research needs to consider this two-way relationship and involve the psychological factor behind what we want to consume.

It's well worth considering what you are currently consuming and drinking before researching the foods that could affect your mental and emotional health. Typically, keeping a food and drink diary every day for around one week is the most effective way to do this. It works better at the moment you have it if you can write down what you eat and drink.

The more detail you provide in your journal, the more valuable it will be; the time and the average quantities you eat, for example, you should also write down. People are constantly shocked when they look back on what they have eaten, and a significant first step forward is greater understanding.

What To Look For Or Take Note Of In A Diet

A fundamental thing to consider for you would be: is there any food or form of food I eat almost every day or in huge quantities? The foundation of a balanced diet is to maintain a balance between a wide range of foods, where the variety is spread over a period of days. Most individuals consume some foods on most days because they are commonly considered safe to consume. Unfortunately, these may be the very foods that affect your health with a hidden but crippling impact.

It is always a mixture of consuming too much of certain foods and not enough of others, leading to symptoms such as anxiety or depression. An essential part of adjusting your diet is ensuring that you only go regularly with the nutrients your body needs. So, if you cut back on one meal, instead of that, you would typically need to replace anything close to eating. For example, this can mean substituting wheat-based bread for bread made from rye flour.

Foods That Affects The Mood

While the exact cause-and-effect relationship between different foods and moods has yet to be fully understood, many people have found that they can relate specific foods to how they feel by eating (or not eating). Alcohol, sugar, caffeine, chocolate, wheat (such as bread, cookies, and cakes), dairy products (such as cheese), certain artificial additives (or E numbers), and hydrogenated fats are among the foods and beverages that most frequently trigger problems.

Other foods widely consumed, such as yeast, maize, eggs, oranges, soy, and tomatoes, may also cause symptoms in some people. Essential improvements in various mental health conditions will result from changes in what we eat. The following changes have been reported: mood fluctuations, anxiety, panic attacks, cravings or food addictions, depression (including postnatal depression), irritable or violent feelings, focus, memory issues, premenstrual syndrome (PMS), obsessive-compulsive feelings, eating disorders, psychotic episodes, sleeplessness, exhaustion, behavioral and learning disorders, and se (SAD).

To feel healthy, which foods do you need to eat?

For a balanced mind and body, water is the most vital material. It is easy to miss drinking the necessary six to eight glasses a day, which is a low-cost, convenient, self-help measure that can improve how we feel, both mentally and physically, quickly.

The nutrients required to nourish the mind and body are given by consuming at least five daily portions of fresh fruit and vegetables (organically grown, if possible). (One part equals a handful or so.)

It's best not to miss breakfast, keep your meals regularly, and choose foods that slowly release energy, including oats and unrefined whole grains. Some protein foods, such as beef, fish, beans, eggs, cheese, nuts, or seeds, are also essential to eat daily.

These eating habits and supplying nutrients help reduce the adverse effects of fluctuating blood sugar levels, including irritability, low concentration, exhaustion, depression, and food cravings. For the development and healthy functioning of the brain, essential fatty acids, especially the omega-3 type found in oil-rich fish such as mackerel and sardines, linseeds (flax), hemp seeds, and their oils, are vital.

There are also significant 'good mood' nutrients in other seeds and nuts, such as sunflower seeds, pumpkin seeds, brazil nuts, and walnuts.

An example of putting these guidelines into effect is The Mind Meal. To draw attention to the essential relationship between food and mood, this was launched by the mind. It shows what can be achieved for emotional and mental health with some positive mood foods commonly recommended as beneficial. Information about the Mind Meal and other nutritious recipes and foods is available under 'Treatments' in the 'How can we help you' section of mind's website.

How To Go About Changing A Diet

It is probably easier if you start by making improvements slowly, one at a time, and only for a trial period. It takes a bit of effort and time to change what you eat; trying out new and different foods can mean you need to shop in new places. Hopefully, you will enjoy making these improvements and find them a positive experience.

Smaller improvements implemented one at a time, should you find them helpful, are easier to handle and keep up. You need to make more than one shift at a time to be able to tell what an impact is having. Some modifications can even be unnecessary, but once you try, you will know. It is possible to extend this step-by-step approach later, and it could be helpful to maintain a food and mood diary.

Sometimes, just for the first few days, a shift in the diet causes some unwanted side effects. For example, if people suddenly stop drinking coffee, they can get signs of withdrawal, such as headaches, which begin to clear up after a few days, when they begin to feel much better. If you cut down gradually, as if you were weaning yourself from a medication, symptoms such as these can be minimized. Certain costs are associated with making improvements to what you consume, but they can be rewarded by substantial mental and physical health benefits.

Supplements And Nutritional Information

A healthy and varied diet of health-supporting foods is the best source of vitamins and minerals; however, you might need to

With extra nutrients, supplement your diet. It is necessary to balance the different vitamins and minerals properly and avoid taking any excess nutrients. Nutritional therapists are qualified to advise on the use of supplements and can prescribe safe supplementation levels for individual needs.

Many people profit from taking a good-quality multivitamin and mineral supplement if it is impossible to get this support. It is also helpful to periodically take a fish oil supplement or a vegetarian oil mix containing 'omega-3' oils. Health food stores, pharmacists, and supermarkets sell nutritional supplements, and you might get a prescription for others.

Food Interaction With Medications

Some people want to try herbal alternatives that can help with the symptoms of depression, such as Hypericum perforatum. However, suppose you are already taking any medication before trying herbal remedies. In that case, you must consult your doctor for guidance: some may interact with other medicines, stop them working, or cause additional adverse effects.

Note: it is very unwise to stop suddenly taking any medication you have already prescribed. As they don't suit everybody, it's also worth consulting a medical herbalist about using these herbs.

In certain foods, antidepressants can interact with a naturally occurring substance called tyramine. A harmful increase in blood pressure can be caused by this, which a throbbing headache can indicate. Beans, yeast extract, meat extract, most cheeses, fermented soya bean extract, salted, smoked, or pickled fish include foods containing exceptionally high levels of tyramine (especially pickled herring).

If you take MAOIs, you should avoid stale food or food that may be 'going off' because the action of bacteria on protein produces tyramine. This is especially relevant in the case of foods rich in protein, such as meat, fish, or chicken. Stop game meats entirely. You can obtain a complete list of items from your doctor, dietitian, or nutritional therapist of tyramine-containing foods.

Food Tests On Allergies Generally

If you have classic food allergies, you will probably already know because the symptoms will be pretty fast and dramatic. However, it is likely to have specific delayed or secret food allergies or sensitivities that are less apparent but may be harmful to your health.

The good news is that this form of allergy can be changed and does not need to be a serious or life-long illness, unlike classic food allergies, which tend to remain.

Food associated with delayed or hidden allergies or sensitivities is unlikely to be detected by tests for classic food allergies. Private monitoring for allergies can do so, but this is also costly. Another choice is a special diet called the diet of reduction and challenge.

This is when you completely cut out a food (elimination stage) for about two weeks and then reintroduce it (challenge stage).

A strong reaction to a food you have avoided confirms the dislike of that food by the body and may also be used to diagnose sensitivities to food. With the support of a healthcare professional experienced in elimination diets, this method is best tackled, who can advise you on the full range of foods you will need to avoid and replace.

A rotation diet can be advised, where you consume different foods on different days.

During the phase of elimination, as you give your body a long rest from a meal, you may go through a phase of withdrawal and experience some unpleasant but bearable discomfort. You will then be in a state of increased sensitivity to the food.

You can have an exaggerated reaction to it if you eat it (either on purpose or accidentally), which some people find difficult to cope with. An experienced professional in the healthcare sector will be able to

To provide vital feedback on these aspects. It is possible to have a delayed answer to a food challenge.

This is when the food induces signs that present themselves just several hours later. If you are unaware of this possibility, it is simple to miss them or not to connect them with the possibility.

Watch out for the food you are eating again and again; there will be invaluable clinical support. Indeed, before making any significant changes to your diet, it is recommended that you consult a healthcare professional.

5

EATING MINDFULLY (MINDFUL EATING PRACTICES)

Mindful eating is a life skill that can lead individuals to enjoy a rewarding, safe, and enjoyable relationship with food that is easy to understand. It is an ability that can help individuals break free of 'food rules' and start embracing safe, versatile, and comfortable eating habits.

Mindful eating is not a diet. Mindful eating refers to how we consume, not what we eat.

What is Mindful Eating?

It is about concentrating your attention and consciousness on the present moment to help detach from normal, unsatisfactory, and unhealthy behaviors and habits to be conscious.

- Eating with Mindfulness,
- Put clearly, it's the opposite of eating mindlessly.
- The mindful eating approach uses techniques that can help alter, both physically and

emotionally, how we react to food. Adopting a mentality of conscientious eating includes:

- Being aware of the optimistic and nurturing possibilities of preparing and consuming food
- By using the senses to discover, savor and taste, preferring to eat food that is both good and nourishing to the body
- Acknowledging reactions without judgment to food
- Being mindful of the signs of physical hunger and satiety to direct decisions to start and stop eating
- Identify personal causes for mindless eating, including emotions, social expectations, or certain foods.

Why attempt meticulous eating?

Research shows that mindful eating can help individuals regulate binge eating and overeating, enjoy eating, and feel more in contact with the body's internal appetite and sacrifice signals.

Many of us might need to be conscious of why we eat mindlessly. Some common contributors may be:

- Not understanding the difference between eating with and without hunger;
- Don't stop listening to what your body signals tell you;
- Confusing hunger and thirst
- Allowing yourself to get hungry and/or to eat too easily

- Eat an amount that should make you feel complete but not satisfied.
- Eating at a later stage in case you get hungry
- In response to some feelings, eating relieves a state of mind, such as tiredness or boredom.

The mindful eating technique uses methods that encourage sensory awareness while eating to help you become more at the moment. These methods include keeping a thorough journal, eating more slowly, focusing on the act of eating rather than watching TV or reading, and making thoughtful food purchases and preparations.

We are conditioned to base our eating decisions on environmental cues (such as the time of day, the availability of particular foods, convenience, to sate our boredom, out of habit, to finish our plate, or as a reward) rather than in response to hunger, mindless eating is very common.

Mindful Eating Strategies

Mindful eating strategies can help decrease the risk of binge eating. These include:

1. Every 2-3 hours, consume small or moderate food.

2. Asking a few fundamental questions before eating

Am I starving? Am I thirsty? What sort of food/drink do I like, if so?

3. Set up a nice place to eat and neatly arrange food on your plate. Don't eat while walking or standing!

4. Being in the present before starting to feed (3 deep breaths)

5. Eat slowly, paying attention to the food's odor, taste, tone, texture, and appearance.

6. In between mouthfuls, bring utensils or food down.

7. Checking in with your hunger signals every few minutes

8. If you are still hungry, stop eating before you feel satisfied and wait 10-20 minutes before consuming more food.

9. Enjoy the meal. You will only be happy if you like food.

You may also like to pursue journaling, a discipline focused on mindfulness. You should use a journaling system or methodology that suits you and that, over a long period, is sustainable.

Some people enjoy traveling with a journal or note-book.; before they go to bed, while others keep a journal to write in. Others keep their machine with a food diary or notes. It could be a list of foods you ate, a poem, a summary of your feelings, or a painting. It doesn't matter what you write.

Yoga, meditation, and walking meditation are also exercises you would like to try based on mindfulness.

Here is an easy mindful eating exercise that you can do to practice mindfully eating at home.

1. Choose one food piece. It could be a raisin, a mandarin slice, a cookie, or a potato chip.

2. Begin by taking a look at the food. Test the shape, color, and texture.

3. Bring the food to your nose and smell it.

4. Place it on your tongue with the food. Note how your salivary glands respond.

5. Be mindful of the sounds in your mouth and the feel of your tongue. Taste.

6. Note how the food's texture varies when you chew.

7. Swallow it now; pay attention as the food moves down your throat to your stomach.

8. Now, tell quietly to yourself the name of the meal.

9. Try to practice a thoughtful slice at least once each meal.

Through the limited success of simplistic models in genetics and neuroscience in describing and predicting eating behavior in humans, the need for a detailed explanation of eating behavior has become necessary. In conjunction with the effectiveness of therapies that normalize eating styles in obesity and eating disorders, the lack of cognitive approaches reveals the central role of eating in coping with these issues. Women have been found to eat at either a decelerated or constant pace in the continuous recording of eating activity and satiety throughout a meal. Unlike decelerated eaters, linear eaters cannot regulate their food consumption when the rate of eating is experimentally increased or decreased, and their level of satiety is disassociated from the actual intake of food. Their reactions to these practical challenges simulate anorexic and binge eating disorder patients' eating habits and satiation ratings.

The general developments of an improved approach for single meal analysis, which incorporates video-derived and intake data, enable the study of the different behavioral components of the meal over time. To compare eating habits between other groups of people, semi-automation, high validity, and reliability make this technique perfect. In decelerated and linear eaters, the chewing duration, the chewing distribution within the chewing sequences, and the pauses between mouthfuls remain constant throughout the meal.

The total weight of the mouth full of food decreases, and in the decelerated eaters, but not the linear ones, the length of the chewing sequences increases over time, demonstrating the essence of deceleration. In addition, the default chewing frequency, quantified by chewing gum, is less linear than that of decelerated eaters, suggesting a baseline disparity between the two classes in the default chewing frequency.

According to some theories, linear eating poses a behavioral risk for the emergence of eating disorders. Although repetitive disordered eating is the cause of eating disorders, it is suspected that the accompanying chewing characteristics may be the mediator of the emotional profile that characterizes eating disorder patients.

The result of eating disorders remains poor, and there needs to be more, if any, impact on widely used treatment strategies. This situation is suggested to have occurred because of the inability to understand that patients with eating disorder symptoms are epiphenomena of hunger and the resulting disordered eating. Humans have evolved to cope with hunger, and anatomically flexible neuroendocrine systems under this evolutionary strain exhibit synaptic plasticity to allow flexibility.

So many of the general neuroendocrine changes in hunger are reactions to the externally imposed food scarcity, and the associated neuroendocrine secretions promote, as required, behavioral adaptation rather than simply making a person consume more or less food. It provides a parsimonious, neuro-biologically realistic description of why eating disorders are emerging and why they are retained. It is suggested that when food intake is reduced, the brain mechanisms of reward are activated. That disordered eating behavior is subsequently maintained by conditioning to the circumstances in which the disordered eating behavior developed for attention through the neural system. Patients are taught how to eat normally, their physical activity is controlled, and external heat is given to them in a method based on this framework. In a randomized controlled trial, the method has been proven efficient.

6

EATING DISORDER AND EATING PROBLEMS

An eating issue is any relationship you find challenging with food.

Food plays a vital role in our lives, and most of us spend time worrying about what we consume. We can often try to eat healthier, have cravings, eat more than normal, or lose our appetite. It is natural to change your eating habits now and then.

But if it feels like food and eating are taking over your life, then it can become a problem.

Many people believe that you would be over- or underweight if you have an eating disorder and that having a certain weight is often correlated with a particular eating problem, and it's a myth here. Eating disorders can affect anyone, irrespective of age, gender, or weight.

If you have an issue with food, you might:

- Limit the amount of food you consume
- When eating, you eat more than you need or feel out of control.
- Eat a lot secretly.

- Feeling concerned about eating or digesting food
- In response to challenging feelings (when you don't feel physically hungry), eat plenty of food.
- Eat only certain kinds of food or adhere to strict diet guidelines and feel very nervous and disappointed if you have to eat something different.
- Doing stuff to get rid of what you eat (purging)
- Stick to strict guidelines on what you can and can't consume and how food should taste, and get offended if you violate those rules.
- The thought of eating such foods is widely disliked.
- Eat stuff that isn't even food
- Be fearful of those forms of food or public eating
- Dream about food and eating a lot or all the time.
- Compare your body with others and care a lot about their shape or size.
- Check, check, and weigh a lot of your body and base your self-worth on how much you weigh or whether your checks and tests are passed.

Difference Between Eating Disorder And Eating Problems

A medical diagnosis based on your dietary habits and medical testing on your weight, blood, and body mass index is an eating disorder (BMI).

An eating issue is any relationship you find challenging with food, and this can be just as painful as a diagnosed eating disorder.

How can your life be affected by eating problems?

Problems with eating are about more than just food; they can be about daunting stuff and painful emotions that you can find challenging to convey, face or overcome—a way to hide these issues, even from yourself, may be to concentrate on food.

Eating issues can impact you in many ways. Maybe you:

- It's hard to focus, and I feel very tired
- Discover that food or food management has become essential in your life.
- Feeling depressed and worried
- Feeling embarrassed or guilty and fearful of other individuals finding out
- Feel isolated from friends or relatives who don't know how you feel or who are angry and disappointed that they can't do anything to help you
- Prohibit social events, dates, and restaurants or public eating
- It isn't easy to be spontaneous, fly, or go somewhere new.
- Discover that your looks have changed
- Discover that other individuals comment on your appearance in ways that you find difficult
- You're bullied or teased about feeding and eating food.
- Build short- or long-term physical health concerns
- You must drop out of school or college, quit work or stop doing things you love.

You can find that other individuals focus a lot on the impact of eating disorders on your body or that they think you have a problem if your body looks different from how it should be. They don't understand how difficult things are for you.

You may also have eating disorders and keep them secret, often for a long time. You may not even be convinced that your diet and eating problems are a 'problem,' as they may feel like just a part of your daily life. Some individuals do not seek treatment because they think their problem is not serious enough or their eating problem is unhealthy.

But it is okay to seek treatment if your relationship with food and nutrition impacts your life. How much you weigh or how your body is built is irrelevant.

7

PSYCHOLOGICAL PROBLEMS ASSOCIATED WITH FOOD

S ome mental health conditions, such as depression, anxiety, or obsessive-compulsive disorders, are often present in many people with eating problems. Food is one of the ways by which it is possible to communicate anxiety, depression, or obsessive-compulsive behaviors. An anxiety disorder associated with body perception, which can also lead to eating disorders, is body dysmorphic disorder.

What Eating Disorders Are

A medical diagnosis based on your dietary habits and medical testing on your weight, blood, and body mass index is an eating disorder (BMI). This segment lists prevalent eating disorders and other diagnoses of disordered eating.

- Nervosa bulimia
- Nervosa anorexia
- Eating Binge Condition

- Another feeding or eating disorder specified (OSFED)
- Other diagnoses that apply to eating disorders

Food is one of the many ways our feelings and anxiety can be conveyed. You may have a highly complex relationship with food that affects your mental health but does not fall into any existing diagnostic categories. More than one eating disorder can also be experienced, or certain signs from each disorder can be experienced.

If you are eating problems are not easy for your doctor to categorize, they will not give you a particular diagnosis. But it is helpful to consider some of the emotions and habits that can be correlated with specific eating disorders, even if you don't have a diagnosis or choose to think about your experiences in a non-medical way.

Bulimia Nervosa-One

You may consume large quantities of food in one go if you experience bulimia because you feel irritated or worried (binging). After binging, you can feel guilty or embarrassed and want to get rid of the food you have consumed (purging).

What you may be feeling:

- Embarrassed and guilty
- That your body is despised or that you are overweight
- Scared of being found out by friends and family
- Anxious or depressed
- Lonely, particularly if no one knows about your issues with eating

- Relatively low and furious, very tiny
- When your mood changes rapidly or unexpectedly,
- You're caught in a loop of feeling out of control and trying to regain control.
- Numb, as if emotions from bingeing or purging are blocked out.

What you may be doing:

- Eat plenty of meals in one go (binge)
- •Go through eating stages, feeling guilty, purging, feeling hungry, and again eating
- •The whole day
- •When you binge, you eat food you believe is bad for you.
- •Hunger for yourself between binges
- •Eat secretly
- Longing for those kinds of food
- By getting yourself ill, using laxatives, or exercising excessively, try to get rid of food you have consumed (purge).

What could be going on with your body:

- You can stay at the same weight or go from being overweight to being underweight.
- You could be dehydrated, resulting in bad skin.
- Your cycles could become erratic or stop entirely if you menstruate.
- Your stomach acid will damage your teeth if you get sick, and you can get a sore throat.

- If you use laxatives, you can develop elongated irritable bowel syndrome (IBS)
- Bowel disorder, constipation, and heart disease

Nervosa Anorexia-Two

This is because you are not eating enough food to get the nutrition you need to stay healthy if you get an anorexia diagnosis. Often people believe that slimming and dieting are all about anorexia, but it's much more than that. It is also related at its heart to very low self-esteem, negative self-image, and extreme feelings of distress.

What you may be feeling:

- Like you can't think of anything but food
- Like you want to vanish,
- That you must be perfect, perfect,
- Like you're never good enough, never good enough,
- Lonely, particularly if no one knows about your issues with eating
- That you lose control by feeding, that you like you need to
- That you're hiding stuff from your friends and family
- It's not just that you are overweight, and your weight loss
- afraid of putting weight on
- Angry if someone is questioning you
- Tired and uninterested in the stuff
- Depressed or suffering from suicide
- Anxious

- A high or feeling of accomplishment from denying food to yourself or over-exercising
- Panicky at meal times.

What you may be doing:

- Decrease food intake or entirely quit eating
- Count all the food's calories and spend a lot of time worrying about them.
- Hide the food or throw it away secretly.
- Prevent unhealthy foods, such as those with significant quantities of calories or fat,
- Read recipe books and cook elaborate meals for individuals, but do not eat them yourself.
- Use medicines that claim to lower your appetite or speed up your digestion
- Consider losing weight all the time,
- Act a lot and have strict regulations about how much you need to do.
- Making food laws, such as listing 'healthy' and 'bad' foods or consuming only items of a particular color.
- Establish very organized times for eating
- Check your body all the time and weigh it.

What could be going on with your body:

- You may weigh less than you should, or you may lose weight very quickly,
- You may become underdeveloped physically (in particular if anorexia starts before puberty)
- You can feel insecure and move slowly,
- You could feel freezing the whole time,

- Your cycles could become erratic or stop entirely if you menstruate.
- Your hair can become thin or fall out.
- You may grow fine fluffy hair (called 'lanugo') on your arms and face, you may lose interest in sex, or you may not be able to have or enjoy it.
- You could find it challenging to focus.
- Your bones can become brittle, and conditions like osteoporosis can arise.

Disorder Of Binge Eating-Three

If you have a binge eating disorder, even if you want to, you may feel like you can't stop eating. Sometimes it is described as eating compulsively. If you have a binge eating disorder, you can rely on food to make you feel better or to conceal difficult emotions.

What you may be feeling:

- Out of sight and as if you were unable to stop eating
- Ashamed or humiliated
- Lonely and vacant
- Highly poor, even useless,
- Dissatisfied with your body
- Anxious and stressed.

What you may be doing:

- Choose meals all day, eat huge quantities all at once (bingeing)
- Eat without really thinking about it, especially when you do other stuff.

- Consuming unhealthy foods daily
- When you feel nervous, angry, bored or sad, eat for comfort.
- Hide the amount you consume
- Eat until you feel sick or uncomfortably full
- Try a diet but find it challenging.

What could be going on with your body:

- Maybe you should put on weight,
- You may experience health issues related to being overweight, such as diabetes, high blood pressure, or joint and muscle pain.
- You can feel breathlessness.
- A lot of you may feel sick.
- Sugar highs and crashes (having energy bursts followed by tiredness) can occur.
- You may experience problems like acid reflux and irritable bowel syndrome (IBS).

Other Defined Disorder Of Feeding And Eating Disorder

A condition that is becoming more prevalent is OSFED. You may have been diagnosed with an eating disorder not otherwise defined (EDNOS) in the past, but it is generally no longer used.

It means you have an eating disorder if you are given an OSFED diagnosis but do not follow all the criteria for anorexia, bulimia, or binge eating disorder.

This does not indicate that the eating disorder is less serious and only implies that it does not fall into existing diagnosis categories. You can encounter any of the attitudes and emotions.

Changes in the body and linked to other eating disorders.

Having an OSFED diagnosis will allow you to access counseling and support.

Some diagnoses associated with eating disorders:

Illness of rumination: You will frequently regurgitate your food if you have a rumination disorder (but you do not have a physical health problem to explain it). The food you regurgitate may be rechewed, re-swallowed, or spat out.

Picaa: When you have pica, you can eat items that are not food daily and have little nutritional value (for example, chalk, metal, or paint). This could be very detrimental.

Avoidant/restrictive condition of food consumption: You will strongly desire to avoid food in general or specific foods due to their smell, taste, or texture if you have ARFID. Anxiety will fill you with the thought of food. ARFID does not appear to be related to body image problems; it is anxiety about the eating process.

What causes problems with eating?

There is no single source of problems with eating, with most experts assuming they come from a combination of biological and environmental variables. It may not be easy to understand why it is, and it has become a concern for you, as the reasons can be complex and confounding.

This segment encompasses:

- Patterns and characteristics
- Challenging experiences of life
- Family problems

- Social pressure
- Physical and mental health challenges
- Biological and genetic variables
- Causes or moments 'at risk'

Traits And Habits

Individuals with eating disorders also share similar characteristics that can make them more

Vulnerable, such as:

Perfectionism-wanting to be perfect and rarely happy with what you've done.

- Becoming really self-critical
- Being highly successful
- Obsessive or compulsive behavior
- A lack of confidence in expressing yourself.

Difficult Events in General

It is possible to relate the beginning of eating disorders to a traumatic event or trauma. Physical, emotional or sexual assault, the death of someone close to you, divorce, or severe family issues may all mean this. Or it may be school or career pressures, such as facing tests or being bullied.

When you go through big life changes, such as puberty, going to a new school, finding out your sexuality, or leaving home for the first time, eating problems also grow at the same time.

Issues From Family

Eating disorders may be exacerbated by childhood experiences or made worse. For instance, you could have started to use food as a way to gain more control over your life if your parents were especially strict, or home didn't feel like a healthy or consistent place. You could have established personality characteristics such as perfectionism and self-criticism if they have very high expectations of you, which may make you susceptible to eating issues.

And whether you were dieting, over-eating or having an eating disorder with other individuals in your family, this might have had an effect on you too.

Pressure From Social Peers

While there are definitely no eating disorders caused by social and cultural stresses, they can lead to them and help keep them going. Movies, magazines, social media, advertisements

And peer pressure means that signals about our bodies and our bodies surround us.

Ideas on how we should look (unachievable). You may not even realize that it is happening, but you may find yourself comparing yourself to these unrealistic images and, as a result, feeling bad about yourself. This kind of social pressure can make you feel like you're not good enough, which can have an effect on your self-esteem and body image.

Mental And Physical Challenges

You can also develop eating disorders if you have physical or mental health problems. It can make you feel powerless to have a physical health condition, so you can use eating or exercising as a way of feeling in control.

As you encounter a mental health condition such as depression, anxiety, bipolar disorder or body dysmorphic disorder, eating problems may begin. Emotions of low self-esteem, worthlessness or powerlessness may be related to them. Having an eating disorder will also lead you to experience these forms of problems with mental health.

Biological Influences And Genetics

Research has shown that your genes can influence whether you are vulnerable to an eating problem that develops.

It has also been found that there appear to be different concentrations of brain chemicals that regulate hunger, appetite and digestion in certain people with eating disorders. For instance:

- Having too much or too little chemical serotonin in the brain can influence your mood and appetite.
- Some individuals may be more responsive to the hormones that regulate hunger and fullness, and this could make them more likely to binge or overeat.

There is ongoing study to find out more about the potential biological and genetic causes of issues with eating.

Triggers Or Causes

Things could help to keep it going after it has grown, but not the cause of your eating habit.

If you have had eating issues in the past or are currently struggling with recovery, you might find it helpful to think about factors that may make your eating problems more likely to come back, such as stressful conditions or going on a diet. These are considered 'triggers' or 'at risk' moments by certain people.

How You Can Help Yourself

It is tough to live with and heal from eating issues. You have to think about food regularly and live in a changing body. But there are also ways you can support yourself to deal with these difficulties. This segment encompasses:

- Speaking to individuals you trust
- Coping with incorrect principles
- Looking for peer assistance
- Handling relapses
- Coping with the comments of others
- Coping with weight-putting
- Change unhealthy habits
- Cope with tough times of the year
- Remaining safe online

Can I think in terms of recovery?

For different people, healing means other things. It could mean you never have to worry or act again about an eating disorder. Or it may mean that you still have them, but they don't happen as much and have less effect on your life.

Your views can also shift over time on how you view your relationship with food and whether you want to recover. You may often feel like you don't have a problem or that your behavior benefits you. Your issue with eating can feel soothing, safe, or even exhilarating. And you may feel terrified of the changes that come with healing. For instance, you might feel:

- Fear of weight loss or putting on
- Nervous to lose power
- The problem of eating is so big a part of your life that you are not sure who you are without it.

Even though you feel ready to try whatever healing looks like, it can take a while to get there. In years rather than weeks and months, you will have to remember. If you've been attempting to heal before or have relapsed, you may feel out of support. However, even though it takes a long time, it is possible to feel better.

Talking to individuals you trust

Eating disorders, for many reasons, can be tough to speak about. But even though people around you may find it challenging to understand eating issues, they will try to help as best as possible.

If you find it difficult to speak, you may write down stuff. For example, writing stuff in a letter will help get ideas out more clearly. It is also helpful to present our data about eating issues to people to help them learn more about them.

Treating Myths and Misconceptions

If you are a male or an older woman, it's more challenging to talk about your experiences. But there are still eating problems for many men and older women.

You will also find that your body changes more rapidly than your mental health. You may feel worse when you start to look healthier, and other people might think you are recovered when you are still finding stuff hard. It will help to keep up the conversation about how you feel with people you trust.

Handling Deteriorations

Going back to old thoughts and behaviors is very common, especially when you are stressed. It may be helpful to recognize periods when you might be more at risk of returning to your eating habits. They may be:

- The times when you gain or lose weight or form shifts in your body
- Go on a diet
- Going on vacation
- Pregnancy and after birth
- High stress cases such as examinations, marriage/civil union, break-up or moving home.

Think about the symptoms of early warning and what you can do to help stop things from getting worse. Signs of early warning may be:

- Eating too little or too much
- Negotiating over food and eating by yourself
- The need to purge

- Fixing and worrying about food all the time
- Check your body or measure yourself more.

In their rehabilitation, most individuals may have failures. But after every failure, you may understand more about yourself and your problem with eating. As part of a long but achievable improvement process, it's necessary to try to be gentle with yourself and accept relapses.

Dealing with the comments of others

Many people don't realize what it's like to have a problem with eating. Some individuals can feel that commenting on your body, your weight, or how much (and what) you eat is okay.

They might think they're saying something good without understanding that you may find it hard to hear. This can be hard to cope with.

For everyone, what helps or hurts is different. Trying to explain to family and family will benefit. Talking to friends about how you feel and what a more helpful or supportive response would be. But it's only sometimes possible to stop people from doing unhelpful stuff. Think about how you're going to handle the stuff people might say.

Temporary Dealing With Weight Putting-On Or Gain

Recovery is not going to mean taking on weight for anyone. But this is an unbelievably daunting obstacle for specific individuals to deal with. Some individuals discovered that these tips worked for them:

- Write down why you want to rebound when things feel complicated, and look at them.
- Take all your clothes that do not suit you or sell them online to a charity shop. Give yourself some fresh clothes in sizes that you feel secure in.
- Try not to waste too much time staring at your body in mirrors or analyzing it.
- If possible, stop measuring yourself.
- Write down all of the healthy physical changes in your body.
- Have a rant or share your thoughts with someone who knows. Speak to other individuals.
- Try not to make comparisons or waste too much time looking at photographs in magazines or online of people.

Dealing With Tough Times Of The Year

Some times of the year may cause complex thoughts and behaviors. Often, these are gatherings that, including Christmas and birthdays, revolve around food and eating with others.

- Chat about how you feel and what will improve things with someone you trust.
- Find different ways of celebrating, if possible.
- Think of things you can do to look after yourself when you find things challenging.
- Understand and agree that there can be moments when you feel out of reach.
- Be patient with yourself, and don't set your goals too high.

Difficulties Of Feeding During Ramadan

You can find that Ramadan creates contradictions between your religion and your issues with eating and recovery if you are Muslim. Some people discover that fasting affects their eating problem-related thoughts and behaviors, especially if they are praised for eating very little. Others learn that iftar makes them feel out of control when dining with family and friends.

If you have a medical condition, although you may be excused from fasting, this may make you feel guilty. Other people might need to learn why you don't fast.

How To Stay Safe Online

You may find that you spend a lot of time comparing your body to others, especially if you have an eating disorder, often without realizing you are doing it. Pictures and photos always surround us, particularly on social media.

Be careful of how you feel when you're online, and change the sites you visit and the people you follow if you need to. Taking a break from social media or changing your lifestyle is okay because it plays less of a role in how you spend your time.

Note that many photographs have been tampered with to make the person look different. And images may have been filtered or photoshopped on social media.

Think of how you treat photos of yourself. Do they make you feel bad, or do you need to change them to hide your appearance?

Think about whether you're following someone whose videos make you feel bad or cause disturbing thoughts. Unfollow them if you can.

Block or prevent any websites promoting eating disorders.

Look for positive communities around food, recovery, and positivity of the body.

What is the available treatment?

Treatment will help you develop balanced and healthier eating habits and help you face the underlying conditions that can cause your eating disorder and deal with it. This segment encompasses:

- Speaking to the doctor
- Free programmes for self-help
- Therapies for Conversation
- Medicine
- Admission to a medical clinic
- Techniques of non-invasive brain stimulation

Speaking To Your Physician

It can be frightening to talk about your eating issues, but if you want help and support, your first move is generally to see your doctor (GP). They should be able to refer you to further resources for specialists.

Self-Help Programs Online

If you are diagnosed with bulimia, a binge eating disorder, or if your eating disorders have similar symptoms, you can initially obtain assistance via an online self-help program. Alongside the program, you can receive brief support sessions. These could be over the phone or face-to-face. If you find it difficult to complete or do not find it helpful, ask for more support from your GP.

Speaking About Treatments

The National Institute for Health and Care Excellence (NICE), which establishes healthcare best practice recommendations, suggests the following talking therapies for eating problems:

Cognitive behavioral treatment for eating disorders (CBT-ED). This is a specially modified type of CBT for treating eating disorders, including anorexia.

Alternative forms of CBT occur for bulimia nervosa and binge eating disorder (CBT-BN) (CBT-BED).

Up to 40 treatments can be given for anorexia, with twice-weekly sessions during the first two or three weeks. It would be best if you were offered at least 20 sessions for bulimia and may first be offered twice-a-week sessions.

You should initially be given group CBT sessions for binge eating disorder. If you do not find them helpful, or if you find them helpful, tell your therapist or your GP. The person would like general counseling.

Family care. This involves working as a family with the help of a therapist through difficulties and discussing the complexities or conditions that may have triggered the feelings behind an eating disorder. It can help your family understand your issues with eating and how they can help you. People with anorexia, particularly younger people, are often offered family counseling.

8

ADDITIONAL TREATMENTS FOR ANOREXIA

These are some additional treatments that may also be offered for the treatment of anorexia:

- Maudsley Anorexia Nervosa Adult Therapy: By helping you realize what makes you addicted to anorexia and eventually learn new coping methods, this therapy helps you move towards rehabilitation. This can be accomplished at a rate that fits you and your requirements. At least 20 sessions should be given to you.

Supportive Health Management Expert: This is not a form of talking treatment, although it may involve talking treatment. You will have weekly meetings during SSCM, where you receive weight gain support, physical health tests, education, and advice. You will also be able to speak and learn more about your symptoms and behavior and key problems you are experiencing.

Focal Treatment in Psychodynamics: You could be given eating disorder-focused psychodynamic therapy if other therapies have not succeeded.

Medicines

There are no medications explicitly for eating disorders, but medicine can be given to address the underlying conditions (such as depression or anxiety). A type of antidepressant known as the selective serotonin reuptake inhibitor is the most popular drug for people with bulimia or binge eating disorders (SSRIs). You could be given antidepressants or antipsychotics if you have anorexia. Alongside talking therapies, most individuals are given this drugs-medication should not be the only thing you are offered.

Being underweight can mean that medicines are absorbed into your bloodstream more quickly, making medicines dangerous or not as effective as they should be.

Your doctor will determine whether to offer you medicine.

Admittance Into An Hospital

succeeded, or if your home atmosphere makes it impossible for you to stay well, you will need to go to the hospital or a clinic.

If you are an outpatient or day patient, you will go home most evenings and weekends. For most of your care, you will stay in the hospital or clinic if you are an inpatient. How long you are hospitalized depends on how much assistance you need to heal.

As an inpatient, you will usually receive a variety of assistance. The hospital or clinic personnel may include:

- The doctors
- Psychotherapists
- Occupational counselors:
- Dieticians

- Social staff
- therapists for families and relationships
- Expert nurses.

Therapy may include:

- Talking Treatments
- Working in groups of other people with food disorders
- Médication
- Re-feeding.

There will be control of your weight and general health. Guidance on buying, preparing, and serving food, dealing with stress and anxiety, being more assertive, handling frustration, and interacting well may be given.

What does 'Re-feeding' mean?

Re-feeding means that food is given to get your weight to a healthier amount, which includes helping you gain weight so that your energy and physical health levels increase.

Relevant foods might be offered to you because they have certain nutritional principles or are particularly effective at helping individuals gain weight. From one clinic to another, how this happens varies. Over a more extended period, some doctors can do this, allowing you to gradually raise your weight, while others may want to help you get back to a healthier weight as quickly as possible. This can be a distressing method, especially if you don't want to gain weight, and it might be something you want to address in more depth with your doctor.

There are only a few facilities for NHS eating disorders, so you might only sometimes be able to access counseling near your home. This might mean going further away to a clinic, or it could mean going to a hospital for general mental health. If you want to know more about specialist clinics, you can ask your GP or health care team.

Private rehab centers still exist. Others can offer NHS clinics similar therapy, whereas others may provide a wider variety of complementary and art therapies.

Being Compelled To Go To A Hospital

Suppose a group of medical professionals agree that you are at risk of harming yourself or anyone else. In that case, they can force you under the Mental Health Act to go to the hospital (often called being sectioned). If your eating disorder seriously affects your physical health, this could happen, and medical professionals are worried that you will not recover without support.

9

FOOD EATING TECHNIQUES FOR BRAIN STIMULATION

Researchers are studying methods that use magnetic fields or a mild electrical current to activate the brain. They can help reduce anorexia symptoms and food cravings, among other things. NICE does not currently recommend these therapies. Further research is needed to see if these methods could be incorporated into treatments for eating disorders.

How other individuals can contribute to help?

This chapter is for friends and family who wish to help those with an eating disorder. You should feel concerned if you think someone you care about has an eating disorder. Knowing how to discuss it with them or how to handle their mood swings can be challenging. You may have tried to provide help already, but you have discovered that the person you're concerned about is reluctant or unable to accept assistance. This can make you feel helpless, angry, and irritated. There is plenty of helpful stuff that you can do:

- Let them know that there you are. Letting the person you're concerned about know that you're there, you're listening, and that you can help them find comfort is one of the most important things you can do. Let the individual know they can speak to you when they are able.
- Try not to get upset at them. They would probably already feel bad about how their actions influence them. As empathetic and patient as possible, try to stay.
- Make no assumptions. People often believe that eating issues are all about body image or appearance, and you can tell what eating problems someone has. This isn't real, however.
- And it might add to their feelings of helplessness if you perceive someone's eating issues in a specific way without listening to the person. It may also make them less likely to share and seek comfort for their challenging emotions.
- Know that it takes time to acknowledge that they have an issue. Patiently be. It can take a long time for someone to accept they have a problem and seek help. The individual you're worried about might not see their eating as an issue. In reality, they may see it as a solution to dealing with feelings of rage, loss, powerlessness, self-hatred, worthlessness, remorse or feeling they have no control over them. They may be afraid of what rehabilitation means for them and their bodies.
- Do not concentrate or comment on their appearance. Know that the weight or presence of someone doesn't tell you how they feel inside. Even remarks such as "you look well" that is

kindly intended can create some difficult feelings for someone with an eating disorder. Instead, try asking, "how are you?".

- Be gentle-you can't compel someone to alter their actions. Trying hard to convince, trick or push someone to eat more or less might make them feel even more nervous about food and afraid of it. This could make them withdraw from you or try harder to persuade you that they are eating better, even though they are eating healthier.

- Involve the participant in social activities. Organize things that do not include food if the person you are concerned about finds it hard to eat.

- Keep meal times as free of tension as possible. Could you not comment on their options for food? Let them get on and consume the food they feel capable of consuming.

- Find safe ways of learning about it. Some say it helps to respond to the eating issues in the third person, such as "that's not you, and that's the eating problem speaking."

- Help them find good data and stop poor data. This may involve searching for resources online while helping users avoid websites or forums that could facilitate unhealthy eating and exercise habits.

- Reading stories and accounts written by people with eating disorders who are ready to think about recovery, such as those included in this information, can also be very helpful.

- Encourage them to obtain clinical assistance. You might offer to go with them if they are concerned about talking to their doctor.
- Agree that it is a long period to recover. Bear in mind that although their body might appear better quickly, they can find it much harder emotionally. Relapses are regular and can be very demoralizing, but when they're rough, you can help by recognizing this as part of the process and being there for them.
- Look after yourself. It can be disturbing and exhausting to help someone with an eating disorder, and it is necessary to note that your mental health is vital and that you deserve to care for yourself.

Therapy For Families

Consider suggesting family counseling if the person you're concerned about is a family member. Family counseling is about working as a family for a greater understanding of the thoughts and desires of each and seeking ways to move forward together-not it's about blaming. Even if family counseling isn't right for you, talking with the family about what's going on will help. It can be hard for siblings to grasp what is going on.

10

FOOD, MIND AND THE BRAIN

Think about this. Your brain controls your thoughts, movements, and other bodily functions at all times. Breathing and heartbeat, and senses, and even while you are asleep, work hard 24-7. This means that your brain requires a constant supply of fuel. Your "fuel" comes from the foods you consume, and all the difference is what's in that fuel. Simply put, what you eat directly influences your brain's structure, function, and mood.

Like an expensive vehicle, your brain works best when it gets premium fuel.

"The "waste" (free radicals) created when the body uses oxygen, which can harm cells, nourishes the brain, and protects it from oxidative stress by consuming high-quality foods that contain lots of vitamins, minerals, and antioxidants.

Unfortunately, much like an expensive vehicle, the brain may be impaired if you drink something other than quality gasoline. If "low-premium" fuel substances (such as what you get from processed or refined foods) enter the brain, it cannot get rid of them. For example, diets high in refined sugars are harmful to the brain. They also encourage inflammation and oxidative stress, in addition to worsening the control of insulin by your body.

A high-refined-sugar diet has been linked in some studies to impaired brain function as well as to the worsening of the symptoms of mood disorders like depression.

This makes sense. If the brain is deprived of nutrients of good quality, or if free radicals or damaging inflammatory cells circulate inside the enclosed space of the brain, further leading to damage to the brain tissue, effects are expected. What's surprising is that the medical community only partially understood the link between mood and food for many years.

Fortunately, the emerging field of nutritional psychiatry today finds many implications and similarities between what you consume, how you feel, and how you eventually behave and the types of bacteria that live throughout your stomach.

The Way You Eat Your Food Influences How You Feel

Serotonin is a neurotransmitter that helps to control appetite and sleep, mediate moods, and inhibit pain. It stands to reason that your digestive system's inner workings aid in food digestion and frequently control your emotions since your gastrointestinal tract produces about 95 percent of your serotonin and is lined with 100 million nerve cells or neurons.

The millions of "good" bacteria that make up the intestine's micro-biome also have a significant impact on how these neurons function and how neurotransmitters like serotonin develop. They safeguard your intestinal lining and guard against toxins and "bad" bacteria; minimize inflammation; enhance how well nutrients are absorbed from your food; and stimulate neural pathways that pass directly between the gut and the brain.

So many studies have contrasted a modern "Western" diet with "traditional" diets, such as the Mediterranean and traditional Japanese diets. They have shown that the risk of depression among those who consume a traditional diet is 25 to 35 percent lower. Scientists account for this difference because vegetables, fruits, unprocessed grains, and fish and seafood tend to be high in these conventional diets and contain only small quantities of lean meat and dairy. The "Western" dietary pattern's mainstays, processed and refined foods and sugars, are also devoid of nutrients. But many of these whole foods have undergone fermentation, making them excellent sources of probiotics.

This may sound implausible to you. Still, researchers are gaining momentum with the notion that good bacteria not only affect what your gut digests and absorbs but also affect the degree of inflammation in your body and your mood and energy level.

Psychiatry of nutrition: what it really mean to you?

Start paying attention to how you feel about eating various foods, not only at the moment but the next day. Try two or three weeks of eating a "clean" diet, which means taking out all refined foods and sugar. See how you're feeling. Then, one by one, slowly reintroduce foods into your diet to see how you do.

They can not believe how much better they feel both physically and emotionally when certain people "go clean" and how much worse they feel when they reintroduce foods that are believed to increase inflammation.

The goods you buy have the potential to help you live a longer, healthier life. Choose the right foods to fill the body with the nutrients it requires to avoid cataracts, infertility, and neuro-degenerative diseases from almost every illness and dysfunction to cardiovascular disease and cancer.

But just as the right foods can help your health, your risk of heart disease, type 2 diabetes, high blood pressure, and more can be increased by the wrong foods (think: processed).

Results emerging from intervention research indicate that diet change (often paired with lifestyle) has the potential for mental health prevention and recovery and may alter the effects of drug treatment.

Dietary intervention studies are useful but methodologically constrained due to heterogeneity in population characteristics, a lack of biomarkers to properly stratify within and across populations, small sample sizes, a lack of medication allocation blinding for participants, and/or a lack of blinded observers.

Your mood and mental health have an effect on every facet of your life, starting with your relationships with others and how you feel about yourself to your physical health. There's a clear link, and vice versa, between good mental and physical health. Stomach issues, sleep issues, lack of energy, heart disease, and other health issues can result from depression and other mental health issues.

In Neurology, a study published on Aug. 25, 2020, looked at factors associated with later cognitive function in 100 older adults with no diagnosed dementia, mainly men. The participants underwent memory and cognitive skills tests and had PET scans to assess beta-amyloid accumulation in their brains. (A higher risk of cognitive impairment is associated with greater levels of beta-amyloid.)

Other variables that are known to affect cognitive performance, such as health history, sleep behavior, smoking, exercise habits, signs of depression, and previous occupations, were also reported by the researchers. Up to 14 years later, everybody was then re-evaluated, with the total age of the participants being 92.

So many researchers found that although some had substantial amyloid deposits, 30 percent had minor if any, cognitive impairment. These same folks have shared similar lifestyle patterns. But they also continued to work several years after the normal retirement age and showed high satisfaction with life.

This resonated with other research with a similar message: a stable brain is an active brain. "While your brain is not a muscle, you might think of it similarly. Without enough exercise, it can become weak and prone to problems," says Lidia Chovwen, a Harvard-affiliated McAlean Hospital neuropsychologist.

One perfect and easiest way to guide against mental aging is by regularly using thinking and brain skills.

According to Chovwen, remaining in the workforce provides many advantages that can help protect and boost brain health.

Working improves social interaction, for example, and is associated with a lower risk of depression, all related to improved brain health. In addition, individuals who continue to work have some additional protection against depression.

The workplace provides the ability to use your mental abilities actively, such as problem-solving, breaking down complex tasks, comprehension (understanding various knowledge sources), and assessment.

As long as possible, older adults should consider postponing full retirement, continue working, and be mentally active and interested, says Chovwen. Many people anticipate retirement, only to discover that they are stuck with nothing to do and nowhere to go. When you retire, think of more valuable things, whether spending quality time with family or pursuing hobbies.

Even if you don't need the cash, a mental boost is offered by getting compensated for work because it validates your worth, says Chovwen. "It shows that you still have value to others and the world and that what you do is important and needed."

Another bonus: you can put your extra money into activities you would not normally do, which enhances brain well-being, such as personal training sessions or stress relief sessions such as massages and holidays.

Consider volunteering if you do not keep a typical job now because of the pandemic. Many possibilities can be accomplished remotely or from home. "Volunteering offers many of the same brain-building skills as a regular job," says Chovwen.

Getting/Having Some General Satisfaction

Life satisfaction, how you feel about your present life and its course, is always a battle for individuals as they age because, according to Cho, they no longer feel a sense of intent.

Volunteering and working will help satisfy this need, but there can be even more overall life satisfaction. Cho says, "It's also about pursuing new goals and having a general enthusiasm for life," Concentrating on personal development and growth can mean re-evaluating your interests.

Cho says, "See this point in your life as an opportunity for new adventure and discovery,"

She recommends revisiting passions you set aside when you were younger or taking on something you always wanted to do if you need a spark. For instance, sign up for college classes in subjects that now stimulate your mind and interest, like history, writing, or science.

11

MENTAL DISORDER AND FOOD

There are several mental disorders or concerns affecting individuals that may be linked to the things they consume. Some of these include:

• Depressions
  • Fear
  • Chronic Syndrome of Fatigue
  • Post Natal Depression
  • ADHD (Attention Deficit Hyperactivity Disorder)
  • Schizophrenia
  • Sleeplessness
  • Pre-Menstrual Syndrome

Experiencing these issues or diseases can also impact how a person feels about food. For instance, a loss of appetite or lack of interest in food may result from feeling nervous or depressed. However, it can positively affect our mental well-being and the symptoms associated with poor mental health by eating regularly and eating more of those foods.

Mood And Diet

A diet lacking in fruits and vegetables can cause a wide range of mental health problems. This is because a combination of vitamins and nutrients is required to keep the brain safe.

Eating various fruits and vegetables can provide a balanced balance of many essential nutrients (at least five portions a day).

It can make you feel tired, low in energy, and unable to focus by not drinking enough water. This is because the body needs about three-quarters of the water and 2 liters (8 glasses) daily to replace missing fluids (more on a hot day or after exercising). Drinking non-caffeinated beverages will keep the body hydrated during the day. Any diet low in Omega three (and maybe six) fatty acids can lead to several problems with mental health. This is because the food we consume and how much we eat influences our mind and body to function effectively.

It is known that eating loads of 'essential' or 'polyunsaturated' fats, such as Omega 3, has a beneficial impact on how well our brain cells function and how well they perform.

Communication with each other and with the rest of the body. Essential fats such as Omega 3 are not formed by the body naturally and can therefore be obtained only through the food or supplements we consume.

Eating plenty of food at least three days a week, such as oily fish, walnuts, linseed oil, and spinach, will provide a good source of omega-three fatty acids.

Waking Up In The Morning With Water

For life, water is essential. Poor focus, headaches, exhaustion, nausea, and constipation may be triggered by dehydration. Since the body is about two-thirds of liquids, it takes about eight glasses (2 liters) a day to absorb missing fluids (more if it is a hot day or you are exercising). Even though they do not feel thirsty, many people suffer from dehydration. And how are you supposed to know if you are dehydrated? A good indicator is the color of your urine! Good has the hue of straw.

You could drink more water if your urine is dark yellow.

It can help you remember to drink enough, or why not keep a bottle of water with you while you are on the go to schedule water breaks during the day?

Here are some ideas to make drinking water more enjoyable, mainly if you do not like the taste. This is good if you want bottled or filtered water, but water from the tap is also fantastic and costs just 1 penny for 12 glasses.

- Attach a lemon or lime slice to give an extra taste.
- Why not apply any cordial sugar-free to a glass of water

By inserting ice cubes made from fresh fruit juice or cordial juice, cool the water down and make it delicious.

- Drink half juice and half water as an inexpensive choice to pop,
- Add a bag of fruit tea to hot water or a slice of lemon to warm water as a refreshing start to the day.

- A perfect way to guarantee chilled water over the next day as it melts is to place a bottle of water in the freezer overnight.
- Make homemade iced lollipops throughout the summer from cordial and water or juice and water and enjoy a superb, refreshing option during the day.

Fabulous Feeling with Fats - Advantages of Omega 3

It is possible to find Omega 3 (and occasionally 6) fatty acids in oily fish and other foods. They include:

- New Tuna
- Herring
- Salmon
- Flax seeds - raw or roasted (also known as linseeds)
- Seeds of Pumpkin
- Flax-seed oil
- The oil of rapeseed
- Hemp oil
- Shrimp
- Walnuts
- Spinach
- Seaweed
- Water cress
- Rainbow Trout
- Mackerel
- Sardines
- Pilchards
- Crab

Eating these foods at least three days a week can be a safe source of omega-3 fatty acids, boosting your mood. Canned fish may also be used. However, check the labels as the omega-3 oils may have been extracted during processing for certain tuna products.

Here are a few concepts to get you started:

- In salad dressings, use oils.
- During the day, sprinkle walnuts or pumpkin seeds over salads or snack on them.
- Substitute conventional cooking oils with those from the above list.
- Add spinach leaves to salads, or why not add them to soups, with Sunday lunch as an extra vegetable, pasta, or pureed-in sauce.
- Have a barbeque for the fish as a transition.
- For lunch, mash sardines and tomatoes together on toast.
- Pick up for free from the supermarket recipe cards for fish.

In addition to the prescribed dietary requirement, supplements can also obtain these nutrients. However, if you are taking supplements, carefully read the labels to ensure that the bottle has an approved kite mark. Alternatively, contact your GP, pharmacist, or group dietician for advice.

Five-a-Day: What does it all mean?

You would have a good balance of vitamins and minerals required to keep the brain healthy by eating various fruits and vegetables. Folic acid, vitamin C, and potassium are high in many fruits and vegetables and are a good source of fiber and other substances, such as antioxidants.

All these nutrients are essential for your well-being, and it will help if you eat at least five portions of various fruits and vegetables.

All these can consist of fruit and vegetables that are fresh, frozen, chilled, dried, or canned and 100 percent fruit juice.

The cost of one fruit portion

For example, half a large grapefruit, a melon slice, two satsumas, three dried apricots, one tablespoon of raisins, one medium apple, one medium banana, one medium pear, roughly a handful.

The cost of one vegetable portion

For instance, about a handful: 3 heaped tablespoons of cooked carrots, peas, or sweet corn, one mixed salad cereal bowl, seven cherry tomatoes, and two broccoli florets.

Can't I just take tablets with vitamins?

Actually not. Since fruit and vegetables contain additional beneficial substances such as fiber, dietary supplements do not have the same advantages as eating more fruit and vegetables.

Here are a few concepts to get you started:

- Chop the fruit and add it to your breakfast cereal, or add it to desserts for extra sweetness.
- It takes just a few minutes to cook stir fries and is a tasty meal.
- Need a snack? For a crunchy snack, have a piece of fruit, or chop the celery and carrots into sticks.
- Drink fruit juice each day with your breakfast.
- Try new ways of cooking vegetables: when grilled, baked or roasted, tomatoes, onions and courgettes taste amazing.

Diary Of Diet And Mood

Evidence is growing that there is a link between the foods we consume and our moods.

It will allow you to see what you eat, how much you eat and what you eat, and how these three items will influence how you feel by keeping a food diary. Writing something down will seem time-consuming at first, but hopefully, you will enjoy it as a process of learning more about yourself and the foods you eat as you get into it.

The Significance Of Routine

Establishing a daily routine will help provide your day with structure and concentration. Eating at regular intervals is important for maintaining energy and blood sugar levels. You might start by writing a shopping list and arranging the week for your meals and snacks. Try working with small snacks in between to provide three main meals daily.

Here are some ideas for snacks that you would like to try:

- Try a small bag of dried fruit and nuts, a yoghurt or a banana for a sweet tooth.
- Melon or pineapple sliced (tinned is fine also).
- A perfect way to get motivation and work towards 5 a day is whizzing up fruit smoothies.
- As an alternative to sugar biscuits, try oat cakes or rice cakes.
- Eating a slow release of carbohydrate food like porridge an hour before bed will help you fall asleep.

Profitable And Friendly Food

Improvements can be pleasant and easy if you have friends and family involved. Here are a few concepts to get you started:

- Sit down for dinner together. It might sound easy, but we don't always sit together in our house to eat. It's a good way to share what's happening in each other's lives and catch up.
- Next time you go on a day trip, pack a picnic or a packed lunch.
- It's affordable, accessible, and enjoyable. If you are in the park, take with you some games to play as well.
- Get the children to cook! Invite some of your kid's friends for a fun cooking session. In the end,

they can sit together and eat their creations
(while you clean up!).

- Get out and about. Find out where your local
markets are, and is there a fruit and veg van in
your area when they run? Can you visit the
Farmer's, Idea Market?
- Is there a food and mood community you might
join that runs in your area? Many local colleges
and centers of adult education run cooking
courses that you can take.
- Do you have any thoughts on other ways of
making eating more sociable? Mark down the
ones.

Here are some top tips and comments to help you get
started, all of which have been kindly suggested by the staff
and volunteers at the HARP Café, a community café run in
Manchester by users of mental health services. For yourself,
check them out.

- "Chop up carrot and cucumber sticks to snack on
during the day."
- I fill two bottles with water and bring them to
drink during the day. I feel much better.
- "You get from drinking water a nice natural
feeling."
- I have fish cooked in my steamer, and it makes it
very quick to bring it in. Spray some herbs, and
it's over.
- A very healthy way to cook food is to use a
steamer, and you can throw almost anything in
there-meat, potatoes, rice-fast! it's."

- Cook some pasta, add tinned tomatoes and tuna and then stir in. Sprinkle with cheese and bake till it melts in the oven.
- "I carry seeds to snack on with me-sunflower and pumpkin seeds are pretty."
- I make a big batch when I cook. Then place some in containers and freeze them, so I've prepared a stock of meals.

Moving to a balanced diet has other advantages. It is capable of the following:

Prevent those illnesses and cure them. Your diet can prevent the risk of developing conditions like cancer and heart disease, and it is also effective for diabetes and high blood pressure care. It can also alleviate symptoms after a balanced diet and help you better manage an illness.

Gain energy while keeping an eye on your weight. A balanced diet will also improve your mood, give you more energy, and aid in stress management. It's a winning recipe for maintaining weight, combined with daily exercise.

Enjoy life. Food is an integral part of events in social and cultural life, and not only does it provide nutrition, but it also brings people together. Cooking fresh and healthy meals can also be an enjoyable way to spend time on your own or with others.

Mental Wellbeing, Health And Nutrition: The Science Behind Mood And Eating

The association between diet and emotions derives from the close relationship, also called the "second brain," between your brain and your gastrointestinal tract.

Here's how it works: billions of bacteria that affect the development of neurotransmitters, chemical substances that continuously bring signals from the gut to the brain, reside in your GI tract. (Two important examples are dopamine and serotonin.)

Eating nutritious food stimulates the development of "good" bacteria, which in turn has a beneficial impact on the production of neurotransmitters. On the other hand, a steady diet of junk food can cause inflammation that hampers development.

When neurotransmitter development is in good shape, your brain receives these optimistic signals loud and clear, and your emotions represent it. But when production goes awry, the mood might as well.

In particular, sugar is considered a major inflammatory culprit and feeds "bad" bacteria in the GI tract. Ironically, it may also trigger a transient spike in "feel good" neurotrans-mitters, like dopamine. Rachel Brown, the co-founder of The Wellness Project, a consultancy that works with busi-nesses to encourage good health among workers, says that that is not good for you either. The consequence is a brief sugar rush followed shortly after by a "that's terrible for your mood" crash, she says.

When you stick to a balanced food diet, you set yourself up for fewer changes in mood, an overall healthier disposi-tion, and an increased ability to concentrate, Dr. Cora says. Studies have also shown that balanced diets can assist with depression and anxiety symptoms. Increased danger of dementia or stroke has been associated with unhealthy diets.

Then what will you put in the cart and on your plate? Here's a short rundown of what to look for when you're in the grocery store next time. At mealtime, you should reach for a combination.

Whole foods

Some studies have shown that hyperactivity and depression may be triggered or exacerbated by preservatives, food colorings, and other additives. Sarah Jacobs, holistic nutritional consultant and co-founder of The Wellness Initiative, says, "So if you have one thing to remember, it's to eat real food," or that's minimally processed and has a few balanced ingredients. Dream of new vegetables and fruits.

Fibers

Plant-based foods are full of fiber, which allows the body to digest glucose or food sugars more slowly and helps you prevent rushes and crashes of sugar. Fruits, vegetables, and nutrient-filled carbohydrates, including whole grains and beans, are fiber-rich foods.

Antioxidant agents

Inflammation fighters are particularly abundant in bananas, leafy green vegetables, turmeric spices, and foods containing omega-3 fatty acids, including salmon and chia seeds. Dark chocolate also has antioxidants and sugar, so be mild.

Folates

Without pushing it to increase the way sugars do, this form of B vitamin helps with dopamine production. Find it in greens, lentils, and cantaloupes with leaves.

With vitamin D

Vitamin D helps with serotonin development, which we usually get from sunlight exposure. But mushrooms are another good source, especially reishi, cordyceps, and maitake, Jacobs says. (Your doctor will also prescribe taking a supplement if you are vitamin D deficient. Members of Aetna may get supplement discounts; check your plan's benefits for details.)

For magnesium

For everything from nerve and muscle activity to keeping a pulse steady, this vital mineral helps. But the food-mood connection is also vital: A mineral deficiency can harm your gut bacteria and result in symptoms like anxiety and depression.

Dark chocolate, cacao nibs, almonds and cashews, spinach and other dark leafy vegetables, bananas, and beans are filled with natural sources.

Foods that are fermented

Probiotics, which are those live bacteria that are healthy for your digestive tract, are filled with fermented foods. Sauaerkraut, kimichi, miso, tempeh and the fermented drink komibucha are examples. (These foods often happen to be high in sodium, so if you have high blood pressure, feed in moderation or avoid it altogether.)

It can take some extra work at first to incorporate good-for-your-mood foods into your diet, Brown and Jacobs say. They recommend cooking chopped vegetables and soaked and cooked beans for a week's worth ahead of time, so some meals are simpler to whip up and as tempting as take-out. Strapped with time? Dr. Corar recommends the use of salt-free frozen or canned vegetables and 10-minute brown rice, quinoa, or whole-grain couscous.

You may also try small nutritious food exchanges, such as white rice, pasta and bread exchanging for whole-grain versions.

This allows the body to increase healthy fiber, which helps with digestion. And for added flavor, select a side salad filled with nuts, seeds and colorful vegetables instead of a bag of chips.

General guidelines on diet still apply. This implies remaining hydrated, not eating meals and being conscious of the intake of caffeine and alcohol. Both can influence your mood or anxiety level directly, Dr. Corar says. "You may want to talk to your doctor about whether you can drink caffeine or alcohol and, if so, how often and how much to stay healthy," she says.

You don't have to suddenly make any healthy shift, Dr. Corar points out. It could be easier for you to take it week by week.

For example, one week you could start by adding more vegetables to your diet, cutting down on sweets the next, substituting some meats in week 3 with beans, and so on. She says, "There's no right way of doing it,"

It's also effective to be mindful of the healthy foods entering your body, especially when it comes to combating cravings. "Appreciate each smell, food texture and taste for each food," Dr. Corar says. And take care of how you feel afterward through the nutritious snacks and meals. For example, some individuals who turn to a more plant-based diet also find that their energy and concentration are maintained throughout the day.

Depending on how many changes you implement, it can take days or weeks before you begin to experience the mood-boosting benefits of a healthy diet. But it can happen, as Cory discovered. Over time, healthy eating helped her to conquer depression, along with daily exercise and medicine.

12

FOOD TO AVOID: FOR ANXIETY & DEPRESSIVE PATIENTS

Juice of Fruit

The whole fruit fiber fills you up and slows down the way your blood consumes energy. You're only drinking nutritious sugar water without the fiber, which can easily hype you up—and bring you down just as quickly. That can leave you hungry and angry—"han." Anxiety and depression will not help. Eat the entire fruit. Drink water when you are thirsty.

Sodas that are Regular

There is no win here for you: it has all the blood-spiking fruit juice sugar and none of the nutrition. Sugar-sweetened beverages such as soda, too, have a direct connection to depression. If you're in the mood for soda, try seltzer water with a splash of juice. Without too much of the stuff you do not need, it will give you a bubbly fix.

Soda diet

There's no sugar, so no problem, right? Exactly not. You may not have the energy crash of consuming too much sugar, but you may be depressed by the diet soda, and it could potentially make you feel more depressed than your sugar cousin would have. It can also be bad for anxiety to get too much caffeine, which so many sodas have.

Toast Breads

Toast, wait! If it was made with white bread, sure. After you eat it, the highly refined white flour it's made from easily turns into blood sugar, which can cause surges and crashes of energy, which can be bad for depression and anxiety. You can make toast with you—and enjoy it, too. Using whole-grain bread instead.

Dressing 'Light'

You may know how to avoid certain sugar-loaded pre-packaged dressings and marinades, also called "high-fructose corn syrup." But what about dressings that are "light" or "sugar-free"? Most get their sweetness from aspartame, an artificial sweetener associated with depression and anxiety. Check the ingredients or, better yet, make the dressing from scratch at home.

Tomato Ketchup

Mostly, they're tomatoes. Oh, yeah, and sugar, a whole lot of sugar. Four grams, to be precise, per tablespoon. And artificial sweeteners in the "light" material could be related to anxiety and depression. Instead, try homemade tomato salsa. Want to kick a little? Add a little piece of cayenne pepper.

With coffee

The caffeine in it will make you jittery and anxious if you're not used to it. It could screw up your sleep as well. Nor does anxiety or depression help. The withdrawal of caffeine will make you feel bad, too. Slowly take caffeine out of your diet if you think it's causing issues. Coffee will make you feel less stressed if you're OK with it, or drink decaf.

Drinks filled with Energy

They may result in abnormal heartbeats, anxiety, and restless sleep.

That's because the sky-high levels of caffeine hidden in ingredients like guarana are only sometimes easy to grasp. Sometimes, these drinks also contain lots of sugar or artificial sweeteners. If you're thirsty, drink water. Want a hit with sugar? Eat a fruit slice.

Alcohols

It can mess up your sleep even a little. Not enough rest will increase anxiety and cause depression, and there may be too many z's that will cause even more difficulties. A drink could relax your nerves and make you feel more sociable. For your mental well-being, that can be healthy. The secret is dosage: the cap is a drink a day for females and two a day for males.

Frostings

It's sugar. Well, yeah, but not all of that. It is also filled per serving with about 2 grams of "trans fats." They're associated with depression. They are also often referred to as "partially hydrogenated oils" in fried foods, pizza dough, cakes, cookies, and crackers. Have your labels been tested? If you eat fat, choose the "good" kind that comes from items like fish, olive oil, nuts, and avocado. Those will make the mood rise.

Sauce of Soy

This one is only for individuals who are gluten sensitive, and it's also in pre-packaged foods such as soy sauce and bread, pasta, and pastries. It can cause anxiety or depression if you're susceptible to gluten, making you feel sluggish and not at your best. Try to check labels and steer clear.

Foods Manufactured

You are more likely to be nervous and depressed if you eat tons of processed meat, fried food, refined cereals, sweets, pastries, and high-fat dairy products. A diet full of whole grains, fruits, vegetables, and fish rich in fiber will help keep you on an even keel.

The Doughnuts

We all love them, and little sweets will help the mood now and then. But you know, donuts have all the wrong kinds of fats, snow-white flour, no fiber for slow absorption, and a lot of sugar added. Therefore, if you have to, make them a treat, not a routine.

Risk Factors For Food Associated With Anxiety

The ups and downs of life make everyone a little nervous. But you might have an anxiety disorder if daily interactions cause extreme or persistent concern. This can result in brief, intense panic attacks, which are sudden episodes of fear or terror. When you have these signs, talk to your doctor.

Some things can increase the risk of anxiety.

Genetics

If you have a family history of an anxiety disorder, you're more likely to have it. That suggests that your genes play a role, at least. Still, an "anxiety gene" has not been discovered by scientists. Therefore, just because your parent or another close relative has one does not guarantee that you will as well.

The Absent Parent Factors

If you lose a parent, or if they leave home for long periods until you're 18, you're more likely to be nervous. It may also result in other family issues, such as crime, alcoholism, and sexual harassment.

Traumatism

The more high-stress incidents you experience before age 21 (such as crime or sexual abuse), the more likely you will have anxiety later in life. Post-traumatic stress disorder may take the form of (PTSD). That is when you relive traumatic incidents in visions or obsessive memories. You might start sweating when this happens. Your heart could also race. If you have these signs, talk with your doctor, and they may recommend treatment and counseling.

Depressions

It's when a sense of anxiety sticks around long enough to affect your everyday life. If your doctor diagnoses you with depression, the likelihood that you have an anxiety disorder increases significantly. If you feel nervous or depressed, talk with your doctor. Some interventions can include talk therapy and medicine for both.

Self-Injury

It's done more frequently by adolescents and young adults, but it's possible as you grow older. It's a way to deal with the memory of an abuse pattern or traumatic incident. You could cut yourself on the arm to distract yourself from mental pain. The behaviors are linked to psychiatric disorders such as depression and post-traumatic stress disorder.

Stress that is Constant

Stressful conditions such as a war zone or a workplace with high activity can lead to anxiety if you are there too long. Continued anxiety about severe illness, economic difficulties, jobs, or troubled loved ones might do it, too. You will help keep anxiety at bay if this sounds familiar if you:

- Let yourself outside
- Keep active physically
- Engage with your family and friends regularly

If you have trouble doing this on your own, get assistance.

The Personality type

Certain characteristics make anxiety more likely, such as:

- Timidity in social contexts
- Critique oversensitivity
- Fixation on specifics
- Moral stiffness

These can also be extreme enough to amount to a personality disorder. Your specialist or doctor can assist you with talking and other medications to work through these things.

Abuse of Substances

If you have an anxiety disorder, your chances of abusing drugs or alcohol increase by two to three times. In stressful social settings, you might use alcohol or medications to relieve tension. The abuse itself could lead to guilt, humiliation, personal issues, and other problems that lead to anxiety.

Speak to your doctor if you believe that you or a loved one is abusing drugs or alcohol.

Solitude

It's not always terrible to be by yourself. And after the loss of a dear loved one, it is natural to feel alone. But it could lead to anxiety and depression or worsen if you feel isolated from the world for too long. That can even further isolate you and start a dreadful loop.

Find opportunities to communicate with friends, neighbors, and loved ones daily. If you ever feel lonely after doing this, talk to your doctor.

Physical Infirmity

Feelings of anxiety are the first indicator of a different problem often. This may include:

- Cardiac disease
- With diabetes
- Problems with thyroids, including hyperthyroidism,
- Chronic Pulmonary Obstructive Disease (COPD)
- Or asthma
- Withdrawal of drugs/medications

Gender

The theories why are not clear, but women are more likely to have depression. Physicians diagnose twice as many women with generalized anxiety disorder, panic disorder, and particular phobias such as fear of flight or fear of crowded public spaces.

13

PSYCHOLOGICAL DEPRESSIONS ASSOCIATED WITH FOOD

The Blues Eyes Beyond

Often, everyone feels a little down. However, if you experience sadness and emptiness and struggle to concentrate, eat, or sleep for two or more weeks, you may be depressed.

This isn't a one-size-fits-all disorder, and it comes in several types, each with slightly different symptoms. Yet it is possible to treat depression, usually with medications, talk therapy, or both.

Depressive Major Illness

This is often referred to as clinical depression, the most prevalent type. More than 16 million adults witnessed at least one episode. Doctors search for at least five signs to make a diagnosis, which affects how you feel, think, and act, including:

- The Grief
- Loss of interest linked to activities
- Selflessness
- Trouble with making choices
- Trouble focusing
- Sleeplessness
- Suicidal ideas or attempts
- Appetite Shifts
- Feelings of shame or loss of value

Depressive Chronic Illness

You may have chronic depressive disorder if you've been feeling down for at least two years. It may be called a dysthymic condition or dysthymia by your doctor. More women tend to have PDD than men, and children and teenagers should have it, too. Their symptoms only need to last a year in order to be diagnosed, and they become more irritable than depressed as a result.

About bipolar disorder

It features emotional highs — mania — and the depths of depression, once called bipolar depression. Not only can these swings impact how you feel, but your actions and judgment, too. That can cause jobs, relationships, and day-to-day life problems. With bipolar disorder, suicidal thoughts, and acts are also prevalent.

Affective Seasonal Condition

For those with seasonal affective disorder, the dark days of fall and winter may be painful for (SAD). The signs are the same as depression but usually arise only when there is less daylight during fall and winter. In America, about 5 percent of adults have SAD. Treatments can rapidly relieve symptoms, such as light therapy or medicine. But as spring comes, they can change on their own as well.

Psychotic Anxiety

This type of depression is very severe. Hallucinations and delusions are among the symptoms. You can be nervous and unable to relax, which can slow down your capacity to think clearly or move normally. A short hospital stay is normally needed for psychotic depression.

Depression After Postpartum

After their baby's birth, most moms feel a little blue. But you may have postpartum depression if those feelings are serious. Symptoms can slip in a few weeks or even up to a year after the baby's birth. Mood swings, bonding trouble with your infant, changes in thoughts and behavior, and worries are normal about your mothering. See your doctor if you think you've got more than baby blues.

Dysphoric Premenstrual Disorder

The cramping and moodiness of pre-menstrual Syndrome in many women are (PMS). But you could have PMDD if you have serious PMS that affects your work and relationships. The symptoms begin 7 to 10 days before your period and go away a few days after your period begins.

See your doctor if you think you have PMDD. Some stuff they'll help rule out. Therapy may include:

- Shifts in lifestyle, such as food and exercise
- Contraceptives by mouth
- Antidepressant treatment

Disorder of Change

Any of the unexpected curveballs of life can bring stress. However, you might have an adjustment disorder that can cause depression, anxiety, or both if it's hard to move forward. You will hear anyone call these "situation symptoms." They start a traumatic event within three months and usually disappear six months later. Depending upon the trigger, they will last longer. Typically, the cure for it is talk therapy.

Depression Atypical

You feel depressed and hollow because of most forms of depression. But if, after good news or a positive experience, yours momentarily lifts, you may have atypical depression. It's not rare, but its symptoms are a little different. Apart from the temporary mood boost, you can:

- Get a better appetite
- Sleep for 10 hours or more a day
- Be particularly perceptive to criticism.

- Let your arms and legs feel heavy, not because you're tired.

Treatment-Depression Prone

Today's therapies work well for most individuals with depression to help them get their life back on track. But up to a third or so of people with the condition need more assistance.

Doctors are looking at why some people do not respond well to treatment. For a little while, some folks will have success with their care, then have it stop working. It would help if you kept seeing the doctor even though your depression is harder to handle.

Depression Sub-syndromal

Subsyndromal means you might have some, but not enough, signs of a disease for a diagnosis. Subsyndromal depression means that you have at least two signs but fewer than the five symptoms that your doctor wants to inform you that you have severe depression. Your symptoms tend to affect your quality of life for at least two weeks to get a diagnosis of this form of depression.

Dysregulation Disorder for Destructive Mood

Children with this condition are typically irritable and have outbursts well beyond expected, although all children have temper tantrums. For some of these children, the prior diagnosis was pediatric bipolar disorder, but their symptoms did not always fit in.

How we feel, think, and act is influenced by what we eat and drink. With the latest data from the Adult Psychological Morbidity Study, one in six individuals

The need for innovative approaches to recognizing and improving mental health has never been greater, having encountered a common mental disorder such as anxiety or depression in the last week.

In order to enhance and promote mental and emotional well-being, this briefing focuses on how nutrition can be effectively incorporated into public health methods.

It explores what we know about the relationship between mental health and nutrition, the risk and positive variables in our diets, and offers an action agenda.

Food is one of the most apparent but known variables in producing mental well-being. The brain is an organ that needs different quantities of complex carbohydrates, essential fatty acids, amino acids, vitamins, and minerals, much like the heart, stomach, and liver. And water to stay safe.

To minimize the prevalence and distress caused by mental health disorders, a comprehensive approach that equally represents the interplay of biological influences, as well as wider psychological, emotional, and social conceptions of mental health, is crucial: diet is a cornerstone of this integrated approach.

Dietary approaches may apply to various societies' mental health issues, but we need to know more. There is, there is

A lack of scientific investment and the conversion of expertise into simple food production and consumption guidance. Food is more than the number of choices and behaviors of individuals.

To ensure that nutritious food is recognized, accessible, and affordable for everyone, public policy is important.

We still need to fully comprehend and apply nutrition's impact on the mental health of the country. Nutrition messages are changeable and inconsistent, and policy and practice changes have needed to be faster to materialize.

There needs to be more progress in accepting nutrition's role in people's mental health through a general lack of knowledge of the evidence base and skepticism about its quality. This is beginning to shift, however.

To make wise decisions that go beyond simply endorsing and promoting, citizens, doctors, and policy-makers must understand the connection between mental health and diet.

Maintaining good mental health, but still having good mental health

Knowledge of the potential for inadequate nutrition to be a factor in stimulating or sustaining poor mental health is growing.

In recent years, integrated mind-body approaches to promoting mental health have risen in popularity, with research supporting the connections between exercise, sleep, mindfulness, mental well-being, and acupuncture.

Dementia, schizophrenia, ADHD, anxiety, and depression are just a few of the mental health conditions that can be prevented, developed, or treated with proper nutrition. There is a growing body of evidence.

In the UK, it is widely accepted that there is a proven link between diet and physical health, particularly for non-communicable diseases like type 2 diabetes, coronary heart disease, and particular cancers. Dietary support for psychological health is underappreciated. This is partly because the partnership is ambiguous, and it is necessary to consider the effects of other factors. Research has also shown a clear correlation between physical and mental health, such as the enhanced association between physical and mental health.

Depression incidence in those with heart disease suggests an indirect correlation. What people eat and how they feel are now directly related, which is more evidence.

The Food Intake General Guideline specifies the proportions of the major food groups that constitute a healthy, balanced diet:

- Eat at least five servings of a selection of fruits and vegetables daily.
- Use potatoes, bread, rice, pasta, or other starchy grains as the foundation of your meals whenever possible.
- Make sure you get some dairy alternatives or dairy (such as soya drinks); select lower choices for fat and sugar;
- Eat some beans, pulses, pork, eggs, meat, and other proteins (including two fish portions per week, one of which is oily)
- Choosing unsaturated oils and spreads and feeding in limited quantities
- Drink 6-8 cups/glasses a day of fluid. These are less frequent and in small quantities when eating foods and beverages high in fat, salt, or sugar.

It can promote healthy neurotransmitter activity by feeding the brain with a diet that provides sufficient quantities of complex carbohydrates, essential fats, amino acids, vitamins, minerals, and water.

It can defend the brain against the effects of oxidants, which have been shown to negatively affect mood and mental health. Evidence of the beneficial qualities of nutrition can be found throughout life.

Healthy food intake has been correlated with academic achievement since a young age, with several studies suggesting that providing kids with

Breakfast enhances their educational success. Several published studies have shown that hungry children act badly in school, finding that when healthy meals are given, fighting and absence are lower, and attention rises.

According to research, maintaining the brain's natural defense mechanisms by eating a diet high in essential fatty acids and low in saturated fats as we age prevents memory loss and other cognitive disorders from arising.

Vegetables and berries

In England, a study conducted by Struangles et al. (2014) found that the intake of vegetables was correlated with high levels of mental well-being. The study found that the behavioral risk factor most consistently correlated with both sexes' low and high mental well-being was the fruit and vegetable intake of the person, along with smoking, among those examined.

Acids, Vitamins and Minerals

A variety of essential functions are performed by vitamins and minerals (called micronutrients), including helping crucial fatty acids to be absorbed into the brain and helping amino acids to be converted into neurotransmitters. They play a critical role in maintaining mental health by converting amino acids into neurotransmitters, fatty acids into healthy brain cells, and carbohydrates into glucose.

In various mental health concerns, deficits in micronutrients have been implicated.

For example, unequal dietary intakes of omega-3 and omega-6 fats are involved in a variety of mental health issues, including depression and problems with concentration and memory; and studies have shown that increased intake of these fatty acids may help manage bipolar depressive symptoms. Reports indicate that, even after adjusting for other factors (income, age, and other eating patterns), these fatty acids are associated with improved mental health and a decreased risk of cognitive decline in middle age.

Risk Factors For Mental Health In Association With Food

There are two classes of foods, generally speaking, that can have a detrimental impact on brain function. One party tricks the brain into releasing neurotransmitters that we might lack, triggering a temporary mood shift (such as caffeine and chocolate);

One group harms the brain by preventing other foods (like saturated fats like butter, lard, and palm oil) from becoming the nutrients it needs.

Eating processed foodstuffs and additives

A systematic study conducted by O'Sheil et al. (2012) revealed that unhelpful dietary habits (including increased saturated food intake) fat, refined carbohydrates, and processed food products) are related in children and adolescents to poorer mental health. Beyeru and Payine (2016) discovered that people with a bipolar disorder diagnosis appear to have a diet of poorer consistency, high in sugar, fat, and carbohydrates.

An analysis of the shifting diets of people living in the Artic and SubArtic regions showed that depression levels were increasing at the same time that conventional diets were discarded and replaced by more refined foods, which were high in Essential Fatty Acids.

14

FOOD & MENTAL HEALTH PROBLEMS

As well as the links, including safe brain growth, between diet and good mental health. There is so much emerging evidence that good quality nutrition can play a role in helping to avoid and treat mental health disorders and recover from them when and if they arise.

A variety of disparities can lead to the emergence of issues with mental health, including the elevated risk associated with poor mental health and socio-economic factors such as poverty.

As will be seen further down, there is a complicated connection between these causes of inequality and poor nutrition.

The upcoming science of syndemics (synergistic epidemics) considers "co-morbid health conditions exacerbated by their social, political, environmental and political environment." This provides a conceptual framework that will aid in our comprehension of the "synergy" between the "epidemics" of obesity and mental health problems as well as the actions we must take to alter the conditions that could lead to them developing into significant public health issues.

Poor physical fitness

A risk factor for having mental health issues is poor physical health. Significant physical health conditions, like coronary heart disease, certain cancers, osteoporosis, and dental disorders, have also been directly linked to improvements in food production methods, such as fermentation, the use of additives, and industrialized farming.

The Poverty Factor

Various psychological, social, cultural, and economic factors provide the context for our decisions about what and how we eat. For both mental health and diet, poverty is a major risk factor.

The dynamic and cumulative effect on the quality of nutrition of poverty and mental health issues is influenced by: income, knowledge and skills, food availability and quality, time, health, and convenience.

There is a socio-economic gradient in the quality of a person's diet, household, and society. Although higher-quality diets are correlated with higher income, nutrient-poor, energy-dense diets are more commonly eaten by people with lower socio-economic status and more restricted economic means.

Household income and socio-economic status affect decisions on what people eat, and as household income declines, this becomes an increasingly important factor. Upon receipt of legislative benefits, people living in households eat fewer portions of fruit and vegetables than those without benefits.

More than 5,400 people were admitted to hospitals for malnutrition in 2012, while 347,000 people were fed by food banks during the same period.

It is important to analyze dietary difficulties' influence on mental health status in these communities.

Co-Morbidity Complexity

Adiposity or Obesity

The relationship between obesity and issues with mental health is complex. Data from a systematic review of longitudinal research in 2010 found two-way connections between depression.

Individuals who were obese had a 55% increased risk of experiencing depression over time, while individuals with depression had a 58% increased risk of being obese.

Although obesity may be the product of poor diets, several demographic variables could influence the course and/or intensity of the mental health association, including

Obesity incidence, socio-economic status, educational level, gender, age, and ethnicity.

It has been suggested that psycho-social factors in childhood obesity are more relevant than functional restrictions and that obese children could be best supported by offering social support rather than concentrating on the diet and exercise levels of the infant. In the 2011 National Obesity Observatory's Obesity and Mental Health Survey', this issue is addressed in more depth.

Strong Drinks or Alcohol

There is a complex relationship between alcohol and mental health. Not only can mental health issues arise from consuming too much alcohol, but they can also lead to people drinking too much. Alcohol, in short, has a depressing effect and can lead to rapid mood deterioration. Alcohol interferes with sleep habits, which may result in decreased energy levels. The central nervous system is depressed by alcohol, which can fluctuate our moods. Some can use it to help 'numb' feelings and to help individuals avoid facing difficult problems.

Disruptive sleep habits, dietary changes, and nutritional deficiencies are also associated with alcohol.

The effect of dietary changes on mental health resulting from alcohol use has not yet been fully understood. Still, studies have shown the significance of vitamin B in preventing dementia associated with alcohol (Korsakoff's Syndrome).

Food/Diet Positions Concerning Specific Mental Health Issues

There is growing evidence that diet plays a major contributory role in various reported mental health disorders. The ties between diet and depression, schizophrenia, dementia, and depression are presented in this section.

Attention Deficiency Disorder and Hyperactivity (ADHD).

The Depression Factor

Depression is the most prevalent mental condition, as stated by the UK's Health Issue. As self-chosen alternatives or complements to anti-depressant treatment, talking therapy and self-management techniques such as mindfulness have been growing in popularity. Interventions that concentrate on the relationship between mind and body, such as exercise either recommended or as a technique of self-help, and new fields, such as acupuncture, are also gaining momentum. Diet has emerged as another thera-peutic method seen explicitly in the practice of dietitians in adult mental health who work to increase understanding and comprehension of nutrition for individuals with mental health issues.

The ingestion of certain nutrients has been related to the recorded incidence of various forms of depression in various major studies.

A most recent revision investigating the link between low fish intakes by country and high levels of depression among people found that those with low folate or folic acid intakes were substantially more likely than those with higher intakes to be diagnosed with depression.

Similar conclusions were drawn from studies that exam-ined the relationship between low levels of zinc and the vitamins B1, B2, and C and depression, as well as from inves-tigations into how adding micronutrients to regular thera-pies caused levels of zinc and the vitamins B1, B2, and C to decline even more.

Symptoms in patients with a history of bipolar disorder and depression.

Schizophrenias

While a complicated area, several studies have shown that diet can be correlated with schizophrenia's onset and development.

The Dutch Famine Study and the Chinese famine of the 1960s showed that extreme exposure to famine in early pregnancy contributed to a double rise in the diagnosis of schizophrenia in male and female children needing hospitalization. Studies also found that individuals with schizophrenia had lower levels of polyunsaturated fatty acids in the body than in the general population and lower levels of antioxidant enzymes in the brains of people with polyunsaturated fatty acids.

Much other subsequent and further research is now being conducted in this field to establish mechanisms by which diet can act to prevent or relieve the symptoms of schizophrenia alongside other treatment options.

Dementia

In preventing some types of dementia, some studies have shown a positive correlation between low-fat consumption and a high intake of vitamins and minerals. One research on 11 countries' total fat intake found a link between higher fat intake and dementia levels in those over 65s. High vitamin C and E levels have been linked to a lower risk of dementia, especially in smokers, in a long-term population-based study. Other studies focusing on different population groups have also found similar results.

Attention Deficiency Disorder and Hyperactivity (ADHD)

In around 1 in 10 (9.7 percent) of adults in the UK, ADHD occurs. ADHD rates tend to decline with age, with the highest rates of ADHD-positive screening reported in those aged 16 to 24 (14.6 percent).

The advantages of essential fatty acids and minerals like iron have been documented in clinical research. In children with symptoms of ADHD, iron, magnesium, and zinc deficiencies have been found, and studies have consistently demonstrated substantial changes in supplementation relative to placebo, either in combination with standard medicine or as stand-alone treatments.

There are emerging but clear in some instances.

Relations between diet, access to the nutrition of good quality, and mental health status. Much as it took some time to recognize and accept the connection between diet and physical health, there has been a similar trend for nutrition and mental health.

Clinical studies point to the value of diet as one of the jigsaws in preventing poor mental health and mental health issues and promoting healthy mental health and brain growth.

However, gaps exist in the evidence base that needs to be resolved if the policy is to represent the relationship between diet and mental health accurately.

With the new evidence base, there are two principal problems. First, creating a causal (direct) relationship rather than merely a connection remains difficult.

And secondly, there needs to be more research investigating the contribution of combined dietary supplements, typically studied in isolation, with individual nutrients. In addition, the comparison of findings is difficult because of the methodological heterogeneity in studies. The emphasis on single nutrients means that there needs to be clear proof of the efficacy of whole-of-diet treatments.

While the overall prevalence rates of mental health disorders can not be dramatically decreased by healthy dietary intake alone, diet plays a contributing role. It is a modifiable risk factor that low-cost, low-risk treatments can target.

A healthy diet is an added advantage in counteracting certain mental health disorders' adverse physical health effects and some medications. For instance, strategies focusing on improving a person's self-worth and developing self-efficacy can help overweight patients improve their emotional well-being and maintain weight loss.

Nutrition has moved the agenda for policymakers, but, as seen in England, Wales, and Scotland, concern has been concentrated mainly on tackling obesity.

Haven said that, in Northern Ireland, the System for Preventing and Treating Overweight and Obesity promotes the interlinking of diet, obesity, and mental health, providing guidelines that adequately reflect the evidence base. The emerging syndemics (synergistic epidemics) paradigm can provide a starting point for understanding syndemics.

A dynamic relationship between socially functioning contextual influences and the rising challenges of public health and personal distress caused by increasing obesity and mental health issues.

There is an immediate need for policymakers, experts, businesses, individuals with mental health issues, and the general public to understand and act on the role of nutrition in mental health. Parity between physical and mental health must be attained. The general public must be informed about the kinds of diets that will support their mental health, just as food is promoted for reasons related to physical health. It would be equally important to comprehend the mediating role that mental health plays in our lifestyle choices, including our diet.

However, national and local policies may have a larger impact beyond individual acts.

Excellent Nutrition For Mental Wellbeing

We're told from a young age that eating healthy makes us look and feel our physical best. What we're only sometimes told is that healthy nutrition often impacts our mental health greatly. A healthy, well-balanced diet can make us think clearly and alert; concentration and attention span may also increase.

On the other hand, an unhealthy diet can lead to exhaustion, impaired decision-making, and slow down reaction time. A poor diet may aggravate stress and depression and may even contribute to it.

A complementary and integrative medicine doctor with the Sutter Medical Foundation, Maxine Barish-Wreden, MD, says one of the most significant health impairments is society's dependency on processed foods. Instead of nutrient-rich foods like fruits and vegetables, these foods are high in flour and sugar and train the brain to crave more.

The dopamine centers in our brains, which are associated with pleasure and reward, are stimulated by many of the processed foods we consume, according to Dr. Barish-Wreden. To get rid of your cravings for unhealthy foods, you must stop eating certain things.

You alter the brain's physiology when you pull added sugars and processed carbohydrates from your diet.

Depression and Stress

Inflammation in the body and brain can result from sugar and processed foods, leading to mood disorders, including anxiety and depression. It is always processed foods that we reach for in search of a fast pick-me-up when we feel anxious or depressed. A cup of coffee is available for a full breakfast during busy or stressful hours, and fresh fruit and vegetables are replaced with high-fat, high-calorie fast food. A pint of ice cream becomes dinner when you feel down (or skip dinner altogether).

When stressed or depressed, people frequently eat excessively or insufficiently. According to the American Dietetic Association. Feed too much, and you struggle with weight gain and sluggishness. Eating too little and the resultant fatigue makes this a tough habit to break. In this case, bad dieting worsens matters during stress and depression. This cycle is vicious, but it is possible to conquer it.

Concentrate on eating plenty of fruits and vegetables and foods high in omega-3 fatty acids, such as salmon, on improving your mental health. In particular, dark green leafy vegetables are brain-protective.

Seeds, nuts, and legumes, such as lentils and beans, are also excellent foods for the brain. Dr. Barish-Wreden says a balanced diet can be more effective than prescription drugs to relieve depression.

"Studies have shown a 40 to 60 percent reduction in depression when people eat the right foods, which is a better result than most drugs," Dr. Barish-Wreden says.

A Gut of Fitness

Researchers continue to illustrate the adage that you are what you eat, most recently by examining the close connection between our bowels and our brain. Via the vagus nerve, our guts and brain are physically connected, and the two can transmit messages.

Although the gut can affect the brain's emotional actions, the brain may also modify the type of bacteria in the gut.

Gut bacteria create an assortment of neurochemicals that the brain uses to control physiological and mental functions, including mood, according to the American Psychological Association. Ninety-five percent of the body's supply of serotonin, a mood stabilizer, is believed to be produced by gut bacteria. It is assumed that stress suppresses beneficial gut bacteria.

Failure to keep the bacteria satisfied with a balanced diet in our guts will lead to depression, Dr. Barish-Wreden says.

When the gut is inflamed by refined foods such as sugar and flour, including whole grain flour, depression can take hold. Dr. Barish-Wreden says people should scrap their bad eating patterns to fix this.

Reducing flour and sugar helps create a new balanced bacteria microbiome. She says it will also help the gut bacteria grow by incorporating fresh fruits, fiber, fish, and fermented foods.

Eating Mindfully

Paying attention to how you feel when you eat and what you eat is one of the first steps in making sure you get well-balanced meals and snacks.

As many of us need to pay more attention to our eating habits, it is suggested that nutritionists maintain a food journal.

A better way to gain insight into your habits is to track what, where, and when you eat.

Avoid what you do when the temptation to eat happens, and write down your thoughts if you notice that you overeat when anxious. You can discover what's bothering you by doing this. It can help to plan five or six smaller meals instead of three big ones if you under-eat.

Stress and depression are often serious and can't be handled alone. Eating disorders develop in others. Your health can be in jeopardy if you find it challenging to regulate your eating habits, whether you eat too much or too little.

You can pursue clinical counseling if this is the case. It is never a sign of weakness or inability to ask for support, particularly in circumstances that are too difficult to manage alone.

Food from the Brain

Your brain and nervous system rely on nutrition to create new proteins, cells, and tissues. Your body needs a range of carbohydrates, proteins, and minerals to function effectively. Nutritionists recommend consuming meals and snacks containing various ingredients instead of eating the same meals daily to get all the nutrients that support mental functioning.

The top three foods to implement into a balanced mental diet are here:

1. Complex carbohydrates, like brown rice and starchy vegetables, will give you energy. More nutritious value is given to quinoa, millet, beets, and sweet potatoes and will keep you happy longer than the essential carbohydrates found in sugar and candy.

2. Lean proteins also provide energy that enables your body to think and respond rapidly. Chicken, beef, fish, eggs, soybeans, nuts, and seeds are healthy protein sources.

3. Fatty acids are necessary for your brain and nervous system to function correctly. They can be found in fish, poultry, eggs, flax seeds, and nuts.

Tips on Balanced Eating against Mental difficulties

Steer clear of snack foods that are refined, such as potato chips, which can hinder your ability to focus. Pass up sugar-filled foods, such as sweets and soft drinks, with energy levels contributing to ups and downs.

Consume plenty of good fats, such as coconut oil, avocado, and olive oil. This will help the working of your brain.

When you feel hungry, eat something healthy like fruit, nuts, hard-boiled eggs, baked sweet potatoes, or edamame. Compared to packaged goods, this will give you more energy.

Create and stick to a balanced shopping list. Don't shop when you're hungry, as you will be more likely to make purchases of unhealthy impulses. Care about where you are feeding and when. Avoid eating while watching TV, which may cause you to overeat and distract you. Find a spot to sit down, relax and notice what you're eating instead. Slowly chew. Savor the texture and taste.

Further Information On Mental And Mindful Eating

It's easy to eat in our food-rich culture without thinking about it. Many mindlessly snack when watching television, working on the computer, or driving. Instead of eating when stressed, frustrated, bored, or sad, some of us eat food when we're not hungry. This lack of understanding can lead to unwanted weight gain and feelings of remorse.

Caren Landy, the Palor Alto Medical Foundation's Director of adult weight loss services, says many people are trying to match their food consumption with their physiological need for nutrition. One way to deal with this during the eating process is to be more conscious and aware.

"We don't always fully appreciate and savor the bites we take, so we end up taking more and more bites to achieve a certain level of satisfaction," says Handy. "You can take back control of what you eat when you eat and how much you eat by mindfully approaching your food intake."

To make improvements, here's what you need to know.

Honor thy Starvation

Keeping your body fed while you are physically hungry may mean that you have to begin listening actively to your hunger and measuring it. When thinking about food, use a hunger scale that ranges from being empty to being so loaded that you feel physically sick. Are you sufficiently hungry to eat an apple? Go ahead, if so, and eat the apple. If not, you're not hungry enough to feed yet.

It will take some time to notice your hunger habits, Handy says, and how much you feed for reasons unrelated to physiological hunger.

"We eat beyond fullness sometimes just because every bite tastes so darn good, or we find ourselves eating to soothe emotions or in response to our feelings, boredom, or habit," Handy says.

Feel the Fullness of your Stomach

Be aware of the physiological signs telling you that you're not hungry anymore. By abandoning eating until your plate is clean, learn to feel your fullness. For a satiety and taste check, pause before eating instead. Are you starving enough to move on? Are you feeling satisfied? Is the food good enough to warrant more bites, or are you only eating because there is food?

You will also identify whether the bite of food in your mouth could be the last one before you discover your level of fullness. Do anything to make it a deliberate act at that stage, such as nudging your plate forward or placing your utensils on your plate or napkin.

Take in Food, Take in pleasure

The absolute joy and fulfillment we sometimes forget can be found in the eating experience. Ask yourself, "Really, what do I want to eat?" That off-brand ice cream tub on sale looks promising, but would your favorite premium brand's scoop be more satisfying? Once you've decided what you want to eat, in a friendly setting, be sure to eat without distraction.

To mark the occasion:

Put your food on a special plate. Don't eat it if you don't love it, says Handy.

Savor the moment if you enjoy it.

Focus on the temperature, texture, and taste.

Stop when you're feeling satisfied and whole.

We get a lot more satisfaction when we pay attention to our food, and we become more aware of how much we put into our bodies," Handy says.

Emotional Eating Curb

When depressed, sad, exhausted, frustrated, or bored, it's not unusual for people to naturally turn to highly refined, sugary, and fatty foods. In response to the heart racing, quick breathing, stimulus-overload sensations of tension, how many times have you munched salty, crunchy chips?

According to the American Psychological Association, 38% of adults believe that stress-related eating behaviors led them to overeat or eat unhealthily within the previous month. Of these adults, 51 percent report feeling disappointed after consuming the food. Since raiding the refrigerator, forty-six percent feel bad about their bodies. It's a vicious circle, says Handily.

Emotional eating may be a numbing fix that is initially satisfying. But it's only going to be a temporary fix,' she says. "Ultimately, learning how to confront that cycle can lead us to a place where food once again satisfies food, not guilt-ridden punishment."

It takes time to learn to distinguish between physical and emotional starvation. To help you decipher whether you are experiencing emotional or physical hunger, here are five essential distinctions:

Suddenly, emotional hunger arises; physical hunger develops gradually.

You can crave a particular food, such as ice cream while eating to fill an emotional need or gap, and only that food can fulfill your need. You're more open to a selection of choices when you eat to satisfy a physical need.

Emotional hunger feels like the food you crave needs to be fulfilled immediately, while physical hunger can wait.

When using food to meet an emotional need, you can continue to eat far beyond the point of physical fullness. You're far more likely to avoid physical hunger when complete.

To relieve physical appetite, emotional eating is substantially more likely to result in feelings of guilt than eating.

One of the most straightforward strategies to combat emotional eating is using the HALT strategy, Handily says. Ask yourself the following questions whenever you are tempted to eat: "Am I hungry?" "Am I wrathful?" "Am I lonely?" "Am I tired, am I?" "If you're starving, respect your hunger by all means. If not, find a way without food to deal with your emotions, such as going for a stroll, calling a friend, or taking a nap.

Often, whether it's coping with depression, frustration, or isolation, the need can be greater or more challenging to handle. To help you work through these problems, see a therapist. Handy says that being a conscientious eater requires time, awareness, and practice, but it's worth the investment.

It will take some real work to find out what the need is, but also how to fulfill it," she says, "Note that what you need is less concrete than food.

Does our mental health matter what we eat? Accumulating evidence shows that this might also be the case and that diet and nutrition are vital for the composition of human physiology and body and have essential effects on mood and mental well-being. Poor diet and the progression of mood disorders are inextricably linked, such as anxiety and depression, as well as other neuro-psychiatric conditions, despite the complexity of the factors that determine mental health. This link is supported by growing evidence.

There are widespread assumptions that need to be backed by solid evidence about the health effects of certain foods, and scientific evidence showing the undeniable connection between diet and mental health is just beginning to emerge. Current diet and mental health epidemiological data do not include information about causality or underlying mechanisms, and future research will concentrate on elucidating mechanisms. Randomized controlled trials should be highly qualified, adequately driven, and geared to advance information from population-based findings to personalized nutrition.

15

RESEARCH ON NUTRITION &
MENTAL HEALTH

I f the aim is to boost mood, improve cognitive function, avoid its deterioration, or even have beneficial effects on some brain disorders, like neuropsychiatric conditions such as epilepsy, attention deficit hyperactivity disorder (ADHD), and autism, information in the mainstream press on the relation between diet and mental well-being is rapidly invading our everyday lives.

There is a common perception that mental health nutritional guidance is framed around a strong foundation of scientific evidence.

For many such claims, it is challenging to prove that specific diets or dietary components contribute to mental health by triggering, preventing, or treating disease.

Conditions related to neuro-psychiatry are some of the most significant social issues of our time, and all the data suggest that the burden of mood disorders, in Europe and around the world, cognitive vulnerabilities brought on by stress and psychiatric conditions will continue to rise in the coming decades. In the public health domain, successful prevention measures are of vital importance.

While challenging to conduct and interpret, research on diet as a key contributing determinant to mental health is urgently required.

The brain's composition, structure, and function depend on adequate nutrients, including lipids, amino acids, vitamins, and minerals.

Therefore, it is reasonable that food consumption and quality will influence the brain's function, making diet a modifiable variable for mental well-being, mood, and cognitive efficiency.

In addition, the composition of the diet is influenced explicitly by endogenous gut hormones, neuro-peptides, neurotransmitters, and intestinal microbiota.

Cross-sectional population-based epidemiological studies can provide information on mental health and illness-related nutrients and diets but do not indicate cause, benefit, or cure. Properly monitored dietary intervention studies of adequate length and precision that show beneficial effects for mental well-being need to be included, with some notable exceptions. Due to small sample sizes, heterogeneity within the samples, and the need for biomarkers to stratify within and across populations adequately, intervention studies are also restricted methodologically.

The essence of dietary intervention, a lack of randomized distribution of care conditions, and/or a lack of blinded observers are often difficulties in blinding participants. The minor effects of dietary treatments in healthy adults can make it difficult to identify them. We have cause for hope, however, as the impact of nutritional therapies may be significant under conditions of impaired functioning or illness. Under conditions of illness or specific nutrient deficiencies (or excess) in the diet, specific nutritional needs can lead to disease progression or severity or cause disease growth.

The advent of the modern 'Nutritional Psychiatry' research area offers promise to define which dietary components are crucial for mental health, including psychiatric illness, and for whom, in which conditions, and at which precise dosages these nutritional approaches have preventive and therapeutic effectiveness.

Scientific results that demonstrate the unambiguous connection between diet and mental health are just beginning to emerge. Nonetheless, several studies have identified clear connections between a balanced diet and mental well-being, which may help to influence potential diet recommendations.

Increased consumption of a diet rich in fresh fruits and vegetables, for instance, has been linked to increased recorded satisfaction and higher mental health and well-being levels.

Diet and mental health have been linked in a number of systematic reviews and meta-analyses. Four cohorts and nine cross-sectional studies, for instance, discovered a link between higher consumption of a "balanced diet," which is defined as a diet high in fruit, vegetables, fish, and whole grains, and a lower risk of depression.

The 2nd meta-analysis, which consisted of eight cohort studies and one case-control, related the reduced risk of depression to Mediterranean diet compliance. More recently, a systematic study incorporating 22 longitudinal and 24 cross-sectional studies has provided convincing evidence that the protective impact of a Mediterranean diet against depression can be achieved. Furthermore, a meta-analysis of 18 randomized controlled trials also found that dietary approaches are promising to reduce the occurrence of depression. On the other hand, a recent meta-analysis of cohort studies showed no critical connection between Mediterranean diet adherence and the risk of depression.

However, a significant inverse correlation between depression odds and Mediterranean diet adherence was found when cross-sectional studies were examined. Together, these findings offer a sound framework for further exploring the mental health effects of particular dietary treatments.

The ketogenic diet for children with epilepsy is a popular example of a dietary intervention that impacts brain development. The mechanism is unknown in this case, but decreased epileptic seizures in fasting conditions, when ketone bodies supply the brain with energy, indicate that an altered energy supply may be instrumental. Another example of an elimination diet that avoids cognitive impairment is phenylketonuria. Moreover, studies have shown that food shortages, especially vitamins, affect memory. Vitamin B12 (its deficiency induces fatigue, lethargy, depression, and impaired memory and is associated with mania and psychosis), thiamine (vitamin B1; its deficiency causes numbness such as CNS symptoms and encephalopathy of Werniicke), folic acid (vitamin B9; its deficiency has adverse effects on utero and child neurodevelopment; and deficiencies are associated with it.

Niacin and (vitamin B3; its deficiency causes Pellagra with dementia as result). Yet the role of mild "sub-clinical" or multiple mild deficiencies in the genesis of mental dysfunction is uncertain, even for these deficiencies. For instance, several studies have tested vitamin D's effect on mental health with contradictory findings.

In community-dwelling elderly adults 65 years and older, higher serum vitamin D concentrations have been associated with improved attention and working memory output.

Randomized controlled trials (RCTs) have, but not consistently, given evidence of the impact of vitamin D supplementation on depression during childhood, adolescence, and adulthood; an effect on attention-deficit/hyperactivity disorder has also been suggested. A large proportion of the general population has vitamin D deficiency based on cutoffs obtained from bone health evaluation, which highlights the need to provide definitive proof of its effectiveness in neuropsychiatric disorders.

A healthy diet that is rich in polyphenols and polyunsaturated fatty acids (PUFAs) and nutritional supplements, including vitamins, have been reported to have beneficial effects on mental health, including cognitive capacity, mood, reactivity to stress and neuro-inflammation, particularly in conditions associated with high levels of inflammation, such as liver and elderly diseases.

This emphasizes that it will be necessary to replicate, refine, and scale-up dietary intervention studies to advance nutritional psychiatry to prevent and treat common mental health disorders. There is, however, an unmet need for more randomized clinical controlled trials.

Cooperatively, the above clinical trials offer specific examples of how specific dietary approaches can change brain function and mental health. Discovery of the metabolic and cellular processes that relate diet to brain function in health and disease will be an important future step. We will need to assess if particular nutrients or whole-food eating habits benefit mental health.

Investigational linctus methods will also help to determine the results of dietary treatments; we must make the best use of existing information, including the collection of suitable biomarkers, to optimize our selection of nutri-ents/diets to be evaluated in costly and lengthy inter-ventions.

Diet And Psychological Health And Wellbeing In Adulthood

A lower risk of cognitive impairment has been associated with a higher standard of diet in adult life. In addition, enhanced cognitive skills have been correlated with the consumption of antioxidant polyphenols in the elderly. Another research found that in an older population, improved cognitive function was linked to a Mediterranean diet that included extra nuts and olive oil. A promising posi-tion for nutritional interventions to combat cognitive decline, especially in aging and in conditions of elevated stress and anxiety, is now emerging.

The ability of diet to exert beneficial effects on mental well-being in clinical and non-clinical populations should be further explored, considering that both elevated perceived stress levels in modern-day life and the growing aging population pose significant pervasive societal challenges.

In comparison, the risk of cardio-metabolic disease and cognitive impairment is increased by unbalanced diets. It is becoming clear that mental well-being and cognitive perfor-mance can be affected by the negative effects of a poor-quality diet, which is likely compounded by age.

Interestingly, nutrition, malnutrition, and obesity, in particular, are strongly related to mood control and suscep-tibility to stress, indicating a direct correlation between food, metabolism, and mental well-being. Moreover, a recent cross-sectional study has shown that physical activity can be partially attributed to the correlation between depressive symptoms and metabolic syndrome. In addition, rodent models' data indicates that anti-depressant and anxiolytic effects of eating a high-fat diet could exist.

Nevertheless, there is evidence from both human and rodent models that cognitive impairments, particularly memory impairments and increased anxiety-like behavior, correlate with a high fat/high sugar western-style diet. In addition, obesity is associated with hippocampal dysfunction and human episodic memory deficits, and studies in rodents have also linked obesity with cognitive impairment based on hippocampal. Thus, as it has anti-depressant and anxiolytic benefits, a technique to cope with stress tends to include increased consumption of a high-fat diet.

In the longer term, though, such a diet carries the possibility of being obese, which is, in turn, related to reduced cognitive functioning and mood disorders.

Clear associations have been identified between diet and cognitive and mental health in adulthood, but we need a thorough understanding of the metabolic and cellular processes underpinning these associations.

Nutritional interventions may help reduce the effect of aging and stress on cognitive and mental health, but to date, there have been few randomized controlled trials, especially in clinical populations.

Food For Brain Sanity

Having clear and not-so-apparent sweet things or sweeteners can save you hundreds of calories a day out of your diet and eliminate a product that could flip metabolic adjustments without authorization.

This is how:

For soda and other sweetened beverages, say no. The calories alone are ample justification to avoid consuming liquid candy: 200 or more calories can be filled with a single 18-ounce soda, sweet iced tea, or fruit drink because of the 15 teaspoons of full sugar such as sweetener, generally HFCS these drinks contain.

Transitioning to an artificially-sweetened, 0-calorie variety is a positive move on the path to healthy beverages, such as water, unsweetened iced tea, tea or black coffee, or skim milk, if you're breaking a severe soda habit.

To discover secret HFCS, read labels. Check the list of ingredients for all the processed foods (as well as other sweeteners you don't need, such as rice syrup) that you purchase for HFCS. It can be found in several slices of bread, sweetened yogurts, and condiments. Just buy the labels without them and definitely with the first five ingredients without them.

Flour that is enriched, bleached, or refined. Both three words mean that they have robbed this flour of its nutrients. Yes, " enriched " means that some of the stripped nutrients were placed back.

Look for 100 percent whole grains instead. About why? At lightening speeds, these empty grains will move through your intestines and into your blood, spiking your blood sugar and causing your body other needless stress, raising blood pressure, scratching your intestines and bowels, accumulating around your waist, having no more to say. Switch your white rolls to 100 percent whole grains (6 servings) for younger arteries, improved bowel function, smoother skin, lower cancer and diabetes risk, and even healthier gums.

It is not entirely clear how eating whole grains affects gum health; however, we know that whole grains help make

our hearts and blood sugar healthier. And research on individuals with diabetes has shown that lower levels of blood
sugar may also indicate a lower risk of gum disease.

About saturated fat - the kind found in beef, poultry
skin, full-fat dairy foods, and palm and coconut oils significantly raises your lousy LDL cholesterol and your belt size.
Being saturated

Because of the bile acids your body uses to digest fat. Fat
can also increase the risk of small intestine cancer. In the
small intestine, these acids can cause oxidative stress and
subsequent cancer-causing damage to the DNA.

And small intestine cancer can be extra risky because it
could raise the risk of other types of cancer, including colon
and rectum cancers.

So for your details, the juicy steak you're preparing for
dinner is probably full of this ugly fat chock. We're not
saying that you're going to

Red meat should be eliminated from your diet (although
we would love to) and only eaten in moderation. You eat
four ounces of red meat on your normal day (that's an
average burger).

Your chance of fatal heart failure or cancer, relative to
people who eat just 4 ounces a week, is almost 30 percent.
So if you care about having enough blood to make your
brain work or prevent wrinkles, or erectile dysfunction,
cutting the burger to once a week can mean a lot to you.
And processed foods are much better for you than the
quarter pounder: hot dogs, sausage, bologna, bacon. So,
without giving up the meaty satisfaction, consider cutting
back on beef. This is how:

Oh, do a change. How about burgers made from skinless
ground turkey, chicken, or even soy or mushrooms instead
of beef burgers? The same research showed that people who

consumed the most chicken and fish were 8% less likely than those who ate the least white "meat" to die.

Make sure that your white meat burgers are made from skinless meat. The big difference is there. If the label only says "ground turkey," for example, it probably includes

Skin and dark meat. That increases your saturated fat intake from 1 to 3% to as high as 17%, more than some lean ground beef!

How about salmon burgers or broiled crab cakes for a sophisticated change of pace? Beans of love? Try lentil-almond burgers or chickpea patties recipes (great with a Middle Eastern yogurt sauce). Turn to a meaty mushroom. In studies, tall, dense, and juicy, Portobello mushrooms are classified as satisfying and delicious as beef and make your arteries younger. Use for a "make yourself younger with great taste" burger in place of beef in stroganoff or throw them on the barbecue.

Note that there is no dividing line between great for you and great taste-yes, it takes a few hours to learn how to make it taste great for you, but in years of better sex, fewer wrinkles, and less impairment, few hours will be paid off.

Using "stealth" soy crumbles to make meatless chili or meatloaf. Give them a hearty spin of sauteed Italian onions, green peppers, mushrooms, garlic, and a splash of oregano, and nobody will taste the difference.

Cook it more intelligently. High-heat cooking methods produce cancerous HAAAs, such as grilling, broiling, or pan frying. HAAAs can be significantly decreased by marinating meat for an hour before cooking, cooking it over medium heat, and using rosemary extract (available from several online companies and shown to reduce the formation of HAAs by about 70 percent) before cooking (available from several online companies and shown to decrease the formation of HAAAs by about 70 percent).

Trans fats, many snack foods, and commercial desserts are still pumped into the ugly stuff. Often known as hydrogenated oils, adding extra hydrogen atoms to unsaturated vegetable oils artificially creates trans fats in the laboratory. They have long been a food industry favorite over traditional oils for their improved shelf life.

However, unlike natural fats, trans fats have no nutritional benefit and raise the risk dramatically.

Of death and cardiovascular disease. Like saturated fats, they raise the amount of LDL ("bad") cholesterol in the body. However, unlike recent studies, trans fat is not just bad for your body and your heart; your risk of colon cancer can also increase.

In one study, relative to those who consumed the least trans fat, around 3.6 grams or less per day, people who ate the most trans fat, an average of 6.5 grams per day, were 86 percent more likely to have potentially pre-cancerous colon polyps.

Trans fats seem to be able to mess with the natural, safe balance of bile and fatty acids of the colon and damage the mucus that protects this organ.

For heart well-being, the Heart Association of America advises that no more than 1% of your calories a day come from trans fats. That means if you consume 2,000 calories daily, trans fat does not contain more than 2 grams. Since trans fat is mainly found in packaged sweets, frozen dishes, and fried foods, they will help. Your other choice is to read the ingredients list carefully, bearing in mind that even trans-fat-free labeled items can still contain up to 0.5 grams of stuff per serving.

More Foods For The Brain

Diet of the Mediterranean. People who were the most active and adhered best to a Mediterranean-style diet in their 70s (mostly fruit, vegetables, legumes, healthy fats, and fish) were more than 60% less likely than people who were the least active and Mediterranean-minded to develop Alzheimer's.

From spinach: Seriously, loading up on this green will keep your brain so sharp that you are the one who wins the account of the million dollars, solves the issue of global warming, and keeps doing the crossword puzzle in pen on Saturday. Consuming three or more servings of spinach and other leafy greens (like kale and collard greens) per day reduces the risk of slow cognitive decline brought on by aging by 50%.

Another way is spelled out: Leafy greens will make the brain work more like someone's brain five years younger! To save your smarts, what makes these vegetables so superb? Nutrients that are brain-friendly include carotenoids and flavonoids. Hold extra strength in your spinach by not letting it stay in the refrigerator. If you store it for more than four days after you purchase it, the levels of carotenoids, flavonoids, and folate plummet, making it a wimpier one. Keep it as cold as possible, too, and it will hold on better to carotenoids. Can't you make arrangements to use it that quickly? Frozen buy. After harvesting, it's wrapped so promptly that the nutrients remain locked in.

Low-carbohydrate nutrition: For successful blood sugar management, there's a new bonus: improved recall. It turns out that insulin deficiency, a problem that causes blood sugar to get out of control, is bad for your organs and arteries and can prevent you from getting out of control.

Recall the name of your prom date, what month it is, or who is the winner of the new American Idol. One piece of proof: Later in life, men who had low insulin levels at age 50 had a higher risk of Alzheimer's and other dementia forms. How impaired insulin response bumps the risk of Alzheimer's is not yet clear. But it is clear that the less insulin in the brain, the more the hallmarks of that illness evolve.

Brown University researchers currently refer to this low brain insulin problem (and the associated brain changes) as "type-3 diabetes." Although researchers have not yet demonstrated how to avoid type 3 diabetes, it is wise to do what you can to regulate blood sugar. Although a low glycemic index diet improves blood sugar regulation, brand-new research has shown that a low-carb diet (less than 20 g of carbohydrates per day) is even better. Ninety-five percent of people with diabetes could minimize or remove their drugs on the low-carb diet, while 62 percent of those on the low-GI diet did. Both also lost weight, which is crucial: obesity is also related to the risk of Alzheimer's.

16

WORKOUTS FOR THE BRAIN

J ust breathe. Inhaling deeply brings into your lungs a chemical called nitric oxide from the back of your nose and sinuses.

This short-lived gas dilates the air passages in your lungs and does the same to the surrounding blood vessels so that your body and brain can get more oxygen.

The workout: Activity improves brain function by ramping up blood flow so that oxygen and nutrients, like your brain, get around better in all areas of your body. It also improves the endorphins that will enhance your mood and relieve anxiety and depression are published.

Additionally, regular exercise will help boost your sleep so that you are less tired and irritable, keep your blood pressure in check, and by moving, your digestive tract can normalize your bowel.

Puzzles with crosswords: Pushing your mind slightly beyond its limits allows neurons and dendrites to regrow, so you are brainpower banking.

From walnuts: Even your heart will love them. They help reduce your lousy LDL cholesterol, the sticky blood fat that blocks your arteries and raises your heart attack risk. Often, they are

Alpha-linolenic acid (ALA), an omega-3 fatty acid with cardio-protective properties, is especially rich in (lowers blood pressure).

To cap it off, they're filled with other nutrients that are good for you, including vitamin E, folate, and fiber.

Flaxseed can also reduce blood pressure. Alpha-linolenic acid (ALA), an omega-3 fat, is abundant in flaxseeds. And ALA-rich foods decreased blood pressure significantly in a study, possibly because this omega-3 fatty acid helps relax blood vessels, allowing blood to pass through arteries and to the brain more freely. Even minor blood pressure drops can protect you against stroke and cardiovascular disease.

With coffee: People who drank at least 3 cups daily were 65 percent less likely than those who were less caffeinated to develop Alzheimer's or dementia. In this brew, the amino acid called anine, whether green, black, or long, is believed to help stimulate a part of the brain's circuitry connected to attention span.

Mint. Peppermints: The effective fragrance makes individuals work more thoroughly and accurately.

Tumerics: Researchers found Indians and studies on mice who eat a curry dish or its daily counterpart have 75% Fewer Alzheimer's than North Americans who do not.

When stepping into new territory, everybody gets butterflies in their stomach, and it's perfectly natural to feel sad or blue when something doesn't go your way.

But you might suffer from depression or an anxiety disorder if your grief lasts for more than two weeks or your nervousness or worry interferes with your ability to work.

Two of the most common mental illnesses in the US are depression and anxiety. If you can eat or sleep, they control how you feel and think, making life a daily challenge. Dr. Gabriella Corar, a board-certified psychiatrist and the medical director of Aetna Behavioral Health, says, "If you are totally paralyzed, and that does not allow you to continue your regular life, then it's a problem." Many people sometimes associate grief with depression.

A traumatic occurrence, such as financial woes or losing a loved one, may cause both. And while some of the symptoms are identical, people who are diagnosed with a major depressive disorder frequently do not experience much excitement and do not seem to snap out of it, weeping, feeling sad, or feeling angry. Ultimately, it causes them to withdraw from friends and family, become tired or anxious, and experience a sense of impending doom.

People with depression, which also induces irrational fear, may often have anxiety. Disorders include social anxiety disorder, generalized anxiety disorder, panic disorder, and other phobias.

The Anxiety and Depression Association of America claims that while anxiety is a severe medical problem that should be treated, only one-third of those suffering from it receive medical attention.

The most important thing, whether you have depression or anxiety (or both), is not to ignore the warning signs and to seek support, Dr. Corar says. These conditions can only get worse in most situations if they go unchecked.

Epidemiological studies have shown that diet influences mental health, and intervention studies reinforce this association. Generally or additionally, individuals with established genetic and non-genetic conditions gain from adhering to specific diets, such as lactose intolerance,

phenylketonuria, and gluten sensitivity. Today, several corre-
lations are disputed; obtaining unambiguous proof for a
causal process is challenging. We know nothing about the
particular dietary components that give the person a mental
health advantage. If a strong evidence base for dietary
advice concerning mental health is to be established, this
research gap must be addressed. It is essential to resolve
many hurdles. A mechanistic understanding of:

How diet affects metabolic processes in the gut
(including microbiota).

This impacts signaling from the gut to the brain
(including through hormones).

How diet affects levels of metabolites in the blood and
target organs.

How cells and neuronal networks (neural networks)
respond.

How genetic networks can be used for mental health
diets.

Elucidating the mechanisms and pathways of metabolic
and cellular processes by which diet can promote neuron
tolerance to insults and enhance mental health.

To enhance mental health throughout life, this will help
us decide how best to modulate the composition of diets.

Nutritional psychiatry's challenge is to establish systematic, consistent, and scientifically rigorous evidence-based
research that describes the role of diet and nutrients in
different aspects of mental health. In particular, the association between the exposure of the body to various micro- and
macro-nutrients (depending on intake, bio-availability,
metabolic function, and organ systems involved) and a wide
range of mental health problems (that include, for example,
mood, cognitive processes, and stress resilience).

And it needs to be better described to include direct and indirect mechanisms which modulate neuronal function and synaptic plasticity.

Much time has been invested in setting up large cohorts for nutritional study. Now is the time to mine data and use the data obtained from such affiliates to identify novel mechanistic hypotheses that can be tested using approaches to experimental medicine. Experimental medicine studies create a connection between pre-clinical process investigations and clinical trials, and they employ experimental design in a laboratory setting to ensure rigor and consistent endpoints. Individual eating preferences and food patterns should also be considered as they, independently of depression, impact total dietary consumption and diet quality). Therefore, new mechanistic insights into the relationship between diet and mental health can be generated using high-quality and adequately powered experimental population studies. Interventions that are more likely to work when evaluated in larger RCTs can then be established.

Nutritional treatments are distinct from those that are pharmacological. Drugs work across one or a small number of targets for which drugs are of high affinity, typically below the sub-micro-molar scale. Vitamins are the only known nutrients that can be tested in a way comparable to drugs, possibly because their affinity is in the same range. Most nutrients are absorbed in much more significant quantities than drugs, and their protein affinity is much smaller than that of drugs. They bind and influence many targets because nutrient levels and metabolites reach far higher concentrations. In general, thus, in several organs, nutrients and their metabolites function on many targets.

While several studies have studied the impact on the brain and actions of particular nutritional components or foods, nutritional research moves from focusing on specific nutrients or supplements to learning dietary habits. This is important since nutrients can work together to influence particular functions, and their bio-availability can be affected by interactions between specific nutrients, thereby complicating the identification of certain substrates.

17

DEPRESSION TREATING FOODS

Milk
It's a strong vitamin D source, which can often cause depression if you have deficient levels of this nutrient in your body. One Norwegian research showed that a year later, Vitamin D supplement users had lower levels of depression than non-users. Doesn't milk like it? Raise vitamin D in your diet with enriched cereals, juices, and canned fish.

Turkeys

The standard Thanksgiving bird has the tryptophan protein building block, which is used by your body to make serotonin. That's a brain chemical that, researchers claim, plays a crucial role in depression. In reality, by targeting the way your brain uses serotonin, some anti-depressant drugs function. Chicken and soybeans will give you the same mood-boosting effect.

Nuts From Brazil

This snack is rich in selenium, which helps protect your body from free radicals called small, damaging particles. One study found that it was more likely for young people who did not have enough of this nutrient in their diets to be depressed. The researchers could not claim that depression was caused by low selenium, however. Just one nut in Brazil has almost half of your daily mineral requirement, so be careful to restrict how much you consume. Brown rice, lean beef, sunflower seeds, and fish are other meals with this mineral.

Carrots

They are full of beta-carotene, which you can get from pumpkin, broccoli, cantaloupe, and sweet potatoes. Studies have related this nutrient to lower levels of depression. There's not enough evidence to conclude that the condition can be avoided, so adding more to your diet can not hurt.

Coffees

A pick-me-up that inspires you can be a jolt of caffeine. But some reports say that it could worsen the symptoms if you have postpartum depression or panic disorder. Other researchers suggest a cup of joe, but they're not sure why it will lower the risk of having depression.

Green Leafs

They're filled with folate that needs to act appropriately in your brain cells, which can help protect against depression. This vitamin, also known as B9, is applied to enriched grains like pasta and rice by food producers in the US. You may also use lentils, lima beans, and asparagus to get it.

The Salmons

This fish and other fish are rich in polyunsaturated fats, such as herring and tuna. Researchers claim that they can help you overcome depression. One source of these fats, called omega-3 fatty acids, can assist the use of chemicals by brain cells that can influence your mood. A few small studies indicate that there were higher levels of omega-3s in individuals who were not depressed than in people with a mood disorder.

Dear Reader,

As independent authors, it's often difficult to gather reviews compared with much bigger publishers.

Therefore, please leave a review on the platform where you bought this book.

KINDLE:

LEAVE A REVIEW HERE < click here >

Many thanks,

Author Team

CONCLUSION

I n conclusion, there are several ways to achieve the best shape of your mind and mood. Exercise, healthy eating, and strategies for managing stress, such as meditation or mindfulness, will keep the brain and the body in tip-top shape.

As attitude and mental well-being slip, it will prevent the shift from becoming worse or permanent by doing something about it as early as possible. Treating disorders such as anxiety and depression increases the quality of life, and stress management learning allows for more fulfilling and productive days.

The biggest concern of older adults is deteriorating brain health. The good news is that, for many years to come, you can take steps to preserve your thought and memory.

A healthy diet, daily aerobic exercise, and proper sleep are necessary to keep your brain healthy. But two additional factors confer mental advantages: work dedication and life satisfaction

Made in the USA
Middletown, DE
25 June 2023

33644903R00113